Series on Bioengineering and Biomedical Engineering – Vol. 9

DYNAMICS of the VASCULAR SYSTEM

Interaction with the Heart

Second Edition

SERIES ON BIOENGINEERING AND BIOMEDICAL ENGINEERING

Series Editor: John K-J Li *(Department of Biomedical Engineering, Rutgers University, USA)*

The aims of the book series are to present a publishing forum for established researchers, educators and professionals in the field of bioengineering and biomedical engineering to promote in-depth documentation of new scientific findings, technological advances, and to provide effective teaching tools of the fundamental aspects of the field. Single or multiple authored or edited books, research monographs, textbooks, lab manuals and specialized conference proceedings are welcome. Topics of interest include biosensors, biomedical devices and instrumentation, physiological modeling and signal processing, medical imaging, drug delivery systems, clinical monitoring, tissue engineering, systems biology and bioinformatics, biomechanics and biomaterials, rehabilitation and prostheses, nano and micro applications to biomedicine, biomedical optics, biofluid mechanics, artificial organs and assist devices.

Published

Vol. 9: *Dynamics of the Vascular System: Interaction with the Heart (Second Edition)*
by John K-J Li (Rutgers University, USA)

Vol. 8: *Neuroprosthetics: Theory and Practice (Second Edition)*
edited by Kenneth Horch (University of Utah, USA) and
Daryl Kipke (University of Utah, USA)

Vol. 7: *Further Understanding of the Human Machine: The Road to Bioengineering*
edited by Max E Valentinuzzi (National Scientific and Technical Research Council (CONICET), Argentina)

Vol. 6: *Cardiac Fibrillation-Defibrillation: Clinical and Engineering Aspects*
by Max E Valentinuzzi (University of Buenos Aires, Argentina &
University of Tucumán, Argentina)

Vol. 5: *Biomedical Engineering Principles of the Bionic Man*
by George K Hung (Department of Biomedical Engineering,
Rutgers University, USA)

For the complete list of volumes in this series, please visit
www.worldscientific.com/series/sbbe

Series on Bioengineering and Biomedical Engineering – Vol. 9

DYNAMICS of the VASCULAR SYSTEM

Interaction with the Heart

Second Edition

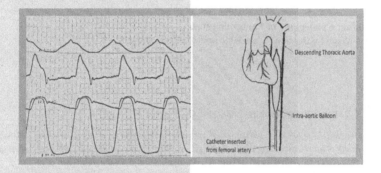

John K-J Li

Rutgers University, USA

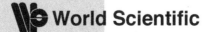

World Scientific

NEW JERSEY · LONDON · SINGAPORE · BEIJING · SHANGHAI · HONG KONG · TAIPEI · CHENNAI · TOKYO

Published by

World Scientific Publishing Co. Pte. Ltd.

5 Toh Tuck Link, Singapore 596224

USA office: 27 Warren Street, Suite 401-402, Hackensack, NJ 07601

UK office: 57 Shelton Street, Covent Garden, London WC2H 9HE

Library of Congress Cataloging-in-Publication Data

Names: Li, John K-J., 1950–   author.

Title: Dynamics of the vascular system : interaction With the heart / by John K-J Li.

Other titles: Series on bioengineering and biomedical engineering ; v. 9.

Description: 2nd edition. | New Jersey : World Scientific, 2018. | Series: Series on bioengineering
and biomedical engineering ; volume 9 | Includes bibliographical references and index.

Identifiers: LCCN 2018010403 | ISBN 9789814723749 (hc : alk. paper)

Subjects: | MESH: Cardiovascular Physiological Phenomena | Models, Cardiovascular

Classification: LCC QP105 | NLM WG 102 | DDC 612.1--dc23

LC record available at https://lccn.loc.gov/2018010403

British Library Cataloguing-in-Publication Data

A catalogue record for this book is available from the British Library.

For any available supplementary material, please visit
https://www.worldscientific.com/worldscibooks/10.1142/9807#t=suppl

Desk Editor: Anthony Alexander

Typeset by Stallion Press
Email: enquiries@stallionpress.com

Printed in Singapore

Preface to the First Edition

This book is the first volume of the Bioengineering and Biomedical Engineering Book Series. As the Series Editor, and to set a good example, I have taken the task of writing yet another book on the cardiovascular system.

The contents of this book extends from *Arterial System Dynamics*, my first book published some fifteen years ago, to distinctly different regimes of the microcirculation and the venous system, as well as the assisted circulation.

The vascular system is indeed so vast, that a binocular vision is often needed to unravel the mystery of the many concurrent interactions occurring at different sites of the vascular tree. This becomes more challenging with the imposition of studying its dynamic phenomena. *The Dynamics of the Vascular System* is written employing mathematical techniques to formulate the physical principles involved in the structural and functional correlates of the underlying physiology. The intriguing control and geometric perspectives are also included wherever possible. The book also serves as a companion text to *The Arterial Circulation: Physical Principles and Clinical Applications*.

Selected topics and references are provided, so that I and the readers are not overwhelmed by the otherwise exhaustive presentations of the many observed phenomena and the subsequent diverse interpretations of their origins and mechanisms.

I hope professionals and students in the field of bioengineering and biomedical engineering, biomathematics, biophysics, cardiovascular physiology and medicine will find this book a relevant source of reference. Much of the work is the culmination of my three decades of learning, experimenting and investigation. I am aware that there are other works of notable items and newer advances which I have not yet included in this book. I will continue to learn more of them. Finally, I like to thank those who have contributed to the completion of this book.

John Kong-Jiann Li
New Jersey, USA

Preface to the Second Edition

This book was originally published in 2004 as the first volume of the *Bioengineering and Biomedical Engineering Book Series*. A decade has quickly passed, together with the many advances in the sciences, medicine and technology. I decided to take up the task to update some of the materials for this second edition, while preserving the fundamental concepts of the original text.

The contents of this second edition include explicitly a chapter on the Interaction of the Heart and the Arterial System. This topic was supported by the National Science Foundation that I began working on right after completing my doctorate at the University of Pennsylvania four decades ago with the late Professor Abraham Noordergraaf. This chapter includes basic cardiac muscle mechanics, the contractile function of the heart and its dependence on the operating relations with the vascular system under normal and heart failure conditions, with emphasis on their dynamic interaction. Examples of mechanical cardiac assist devices and drug treatment are also included.

This second edition continues to emphasize on quantitative treatment of the vascular system by analyzing the structural and functional correlates of the underlying physiology. This may purposefully overlook some of the clinical aspects in terms of diagnosis and treatment efficacies of certain cardiovascular diseases. Similar to the first edition, rather than being exhaustive, only selected topics and references are provided. In this regard, worthwhile publications from some investigators may not have been included.

I hope many of the cardiovascular scientists, researchers and clinicians, as well as students will continue to find this book a useful reference. I like to thank those who have contributed to the completion of this book.

John Kong-Jiann Li
New Jersey, USA

About the Author

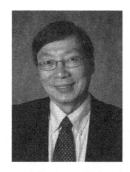John K-J. Li obtained his Ph.D. in Bioengineering from the University of Pennsylvania and has been a Distinguished Professor of Biomedical Engineering at Rutgers University since 1998. He has been an elected Fellow of the American Institute for Medical and Biological Engineering, the American Colleges of Cardiology, the American College of Angiology, and the Academy of Medicine of New Jersey. He is also the Founding Editor-in-chief of Springer's *Cardiovascular Engineering* and *Bioengineering and Biomedical Engineering* Book Series of World Scientific and Imperial College Press, and is on the editorial boards of numerous journals. His research has been founded by the NIH, NSF, AHA, and industry grants, with interest in cardiac and vascular mechanics, modeling, medical devices, controlled drug delivery, hypertension and heart failure, neuroengineering, scaling in biology, and comparative physiology. He has authored several books and published numerous articles and is a frequently invited speaker at national and international conferences and universities. He enjoys teaching and has been the adviser to more than 90 Ph.D. and M.S. students and 175 senior design students, and received teaching excellence awards. He is also a holder of several US patents and a recipient of the IEEE Millennium Medal.

Contents

Preface to the First Edition v

Preface to the Second Edition vii

About the Author ix

Chapter 1. Historical Background and Book Contents 1

  1.1 Discoveries of the Circulation 1
  1.2 Importance of the Vascular System 7
  1.3 Newer Concepts...8
  1.4 Book Contents 9

Chapter 2. Vascular Biology, Structure and Function 15

  2.1 Anatomical Organization of the Vasculature...............15
      2.1.1 The Closed-loop Circulatory System.................15
      2.1.2 The Heart 15
      2.1.3 The Arteries 18
      2.1.4 The Veins..19
      2.1.5 The Microvasculature 20
  2.2 Geometric and Mechanical Properties of Blood Vessels.........21
      2.2.1 Geometric Nonuniformity of Blood Vessels 21
      2.2.2 Elastic Nonuniformity of the Blood Vessels 24
      2.2.3 Vascular Stiffness and Elastic Properties 25
  2.3 Functional Properties of Blood...................................31
      2.3.1 Blood Plasma and Blood Gas 31
      2.3.2 Oxygen Saturation Curves and Hemoglobin 32
      2.3.3 Red Blood Cells, Hematocrit and Blood Volume.........35

2.4 Control Aspects of the Vascular System 37
      2.4.1 Control of the Central Cardiovascular System 38
      2.4.2 Functions of the Baroreceptors...................................39
      2.4.3 Arterial Chemoreceptors...40

Chapter 3. Physical Concepts and Basic Fluid Mechanics 43

3.1 Basic Mechanics and Dimensional Analysis..........................43
      3.1.1 Mass, Length and Time System and the Pi-theorem
              of Buckingham 43
      3.1.2 Dimensional Matrix...45
      3.1.3 Biological Scaling and Dynamics Similitude in
              Vascular Biology..46
      3.1.4 Elastic and Viscoelastic Properties of Blood
              Vessels...49
3.2 Frequency Domain and Fourier Analysis 56
      3.2.1 Blood Pressure as a Periodic Function 56
      3.2.2 Trigonometric Fourier Series......................................57
      3.2.3 Complex Form of Fourier Series 59
      3.2.4 Other Aspects of Frequency Domain Analysis............62
              3.2.4.1 Dirichlet Conditions 62
              3.2.4.2 Line Spectrum and Nyquist Criterion..............63
              3.2.4.3 Correlation, Coherence and Power
                          Spectrum 64
3.3 Fluid Mechanics and Rheology 65
      3.3.1 Steady Flow, the Poiseuille Equation and Flow
              Velocity Profile...65
      3.3.2 Bernoulli's Equation and Narrowing Vessel Lumen
              or Stenosis..70
      3.3.3 Orifice Flow and Torricelli's Equation.......................71
      3.3.4 Valvular Cross-section and the Gorlin Equation 72
      3.3.5 Flow and Flow Acceleration.......................................72
      3.3.6 Newtonian Fluid, No-Slip, Boundary Conditions
              and Entry Length 75
              3.3.6.1 Newtonian Fluid...75
              3.3.6.2 No-Slip Boundary Conditions 76
              3.3.6.3 Laminar and Turbulent Flow............................77
              3.3.6.4 Entry Length...78

Chapter 4. Hemodynamics of Arteries...79

4.1 Blood Pressure and Flow Relations 79
 4.1.1 Pulsatile Pressure and Flow Waveforms
  in Arteries 79
 4.1.2 Pressure-flow Relations in the Aorta...........................82
4.2 Vascular Impedance to Blood Flow..84
 4.2.1 The Impedance Concept and Formulation....................84
 4.2.2 Input Impedance and Characteristic Impedance...........86
4.3 Pulse Wave Propagation Phenomena..90
 4.3.1 The Pulse Wave Propagation Constant........................90
 4.3.2 Pulse Wave Velocity and the Foot-to-Foot
  Velocity 91
 4.3.3 Apparent Propagation Constant and Transfer
  Function 94
 4.3.4 Determination of the Propagation Constant
  and Frequency Dependent Pulse Wave Velocity...........98
4.4 Pulse Wave Reflection Phenomena 102
 4.4.1 Influence of Wave Reflections on Pressure
  and Flow Waveforms..102
 4.4.2 The Reflection Coefficients.....................................108
 4.4.3 The Augmentation Index 111
 4.4.4 Wave Reflection Sites and Multiple Reflections.........112
4.5 Modeling Aspects of the Arterial Circulation..........................114
 4.5.1 Mathematical Formulations of Pulse Wave
  Propagation 114
 4.5.2 Linear Theories of Oscillatory Blood Flow in
  Arteries 118
 4.5.3 The Lumped Model of the Arterial System and the
  Windkessel Model 124
 4.5.4 Nonlinear Aspects and Pressure-Dependent
  Arterial Compliance..130

Chapter 5. Vascular Branching 137

5.1 Branching Geometry..137
 5.1.1 Complexity of Vascular Branching 137
 5.1.2 Nonuniform Branching and 3-D Branching
  Structures 139
 5.1.3 Space-Filling Properties and Modeling 141

5.2   Fluid Mechanics of Vascular Branching.................................144
        5.2.1   Branching Geometry and Fluid Dynamic
                   Considerations 144
        5.2.2   Fluid Mechanics Associated with Atherosclerosis
                   and Stenosis...149
5.3   Pulse Transmission Characteristics at Vascular
        Branching...151
        5.3.1   Impedance Matching and Wave Reflections 151
        5.3.2   Area Ratio Concept..154
        5.3.3   Minimum Local Reflections at Vascular Branching
                   Junctions 158
5.4   Optimization Aspects Applicable to Vascular Branching 161
        5.4.1   Optimizing Vessel Radius and the Cube Law 161
        5.4.2   Optimizing Branching Radii and Angles....................164

Chapter 6. The Venous System...167

6.1   The Reservoir Properties and Venous Return......................167
        6.1.1   Venous Compliance and Reservoir Characteristics.....167
        6.1.2   Structural Properties of Veins.................................168
        6.1.3   Venous Return 169
6.2   Pressure and Flow Waveforms in Veins.............................170
        6.2.1   The Normal Pressure and Flow Waveforms
                   in Veins..170
        6.2.2   Respiration Effects on Venous Pressure and Flow
                   Waveforms..172
        6.2.3   Abnormal Venous Pressure and Flow Waveforms......173
6.3   Modeling and Collapsible Vessel Properties 173
        6.3.1   Steady Flow in Collapsible Tubes 173
        6.3.2   Flow Limitation and Model Experiments...................175
        6.3.3   Pulse Wave Transmission Characteristics in Veins.....180

Chapter 7. The Microcirculation...183

7.1   Structure of the Microcirculation.....................................183
        7.1.1   Functional Organization of the Microvasculature 183
        7.1.2   The Capillary Circulation 188
7.2   Pressure-Flow Relation and Microcirculatory Mechanics......191
        7.2.1   Flow-Related Mechanical Characteristics of the
                   Microcirculation 191

7.2.2 Some Pressure-Related Mechanical Characteristics
of the Microcirculation 193
7.3 Pulse Transmission and Modeling Aspects 196
7.3.1 Pressure and Flow Waveforms in Arterioles
and Capillaries 196
7.3.2 Pulse Transmission Characteristics in the
Microcirculation 198
7.3.3 Modeling Aspects of the Microcirculation 201

Chapter 8. Hemodynamic Measurements: Invasive and
Noninvasive Monitoring 205

8.1 Catheterization for Blood Pressure Measurement 205
8.1.1 Fluid-filled Blood Pressure Measurement
Systems 205
8.1.2 Experimental Evaluation of the Frequency
Response of Catheter-Pressure Transducer
Systems 208
8.2 Noninvasive Blood Pressure Measurements 213
8.2.1 Auscultation Measurement of Blood Pressure 213
8.2.2 Blood Pressure Measurement with the Oscillometric
Method 215
8.2.3 Noninvasive Blood Pressure Monitoring with
Tonometer 217
8.2.4 The Photoplethysmograph (PPG) 219
8.3 Blood Flow Measurement 219
8.3.1 Electromagnetic Flowmeter 219
8.3.2 Ultrasound and Doppler Flow Velocity
Measurement 221
8.3.3 Cardiac Output Measurement with Indicator
Dilution Methods and Thermodilution 224
8.4 Measurement of Vascular Dimensions 227

Chapter 9. Interaction of the Heart and the Arterial System 229

9.1 Ventricular Outflow and the Aorta 229
9.1.1 Ventricular Ejection 229

9.2   Cardiac Muscle Mechanics and the Force-Velocity-Length
      Relation 232
      9.2.1   Structure of Myocardial Fibers and the Sliding
              Filament Theory 232
      9.2.2   Hill Model of Muscle Contraction...............................234
9.3   The Pressure-Volume Curve and Contractility
      of the Heart 235
      9.3.1   Variables Defining the Pressure-Volume Loop...........235
      9.3.2   Frank-Starling Mechanism and Ejection Fraction 237
      9.3.3   Cardiac Contractility and Indices of Cardiac
              Performance..239
9.4   Heart and the Arterial System Interaction 241
      9.4.1   The Concept of Ventricular and Arterial
              Elastances 241
      9.4.2   Dynamic Heart-Arterial System Interaction 246
      9.4.3   Left Ventricle-Arterial System Interaction
              in Heart Failure...248
9.5   Heart-Arterial System Interaction in the Assisted
      Circulation 250
      9.5.1   Mechanical Assist Devices and the Intra-Aortic
              Balloon Pump 250
      9.5.2   Optimization of Intra-Aortic Balloon Pumping:
              Physiological Considerations..254
      9.5.3   Optimization of Intra-Aortic Balloon Pumping:
              Modeling Aspects 258
      9.5.4   Optimization of Intra-Aortic Balloon Pumping:
              Control Aspects 259

Bibliography 261

Index..273

Chapter 1

Historical Background and Book Contents

1.1 Discoveries of the Circulation

That "blood moves in closed circle" was apparently known in the Far East, several millennia ago, about 2,650 B.C., as recorded in the book by the Yellow Emperor of China written in the Canon of Medicine (Nei Ching). Ancient Chinese practitioners customarily felt palpable wrist artery (radial artery) pulsations as a means of diagnosing the cardiac state of their patients. In this approach, the practitioners were able to obtain both the strength of the pulsation to infer the vigor of contraction of the heart, and the interval duration of the pulses, hence heart rate. This seemingly indicates that the importance of the rate-pressure product, now a popular clinical index of myocardial oxygen consumption, might even have been considered pertinent at that time. The supply and demand of oxygenation, as well as its proper utilization in terms of energy balance, or ying-yang, is center to achieving body harmony. Thus, this suggestion of an intrinsic transfer of the energy (Chi) generated by the heart to the peripheral arteries may have been known since antiquity, although the theoretical foundation was not established until much later.

In the West, the observation that man must inspire air to sustain life led ancient scientists and philosophers to toy with the idea that arteries contained air rather than blood. This was the notion originally attributed to Erasistratus in the third century B.C., following the teaching of Aristotle. Aristotle and later Herophilus performed numerous anatomical studies and the latter discovered the connecting arteries to the contracting heart. That arteries themselves contract and relax thus was known in Aristotle's time. Arterial properties in terms of elastic stiffness, distensibility and compliance, as we know now, were not fully described. Galen's (130-200) description of the ebb and flow of blood in arteries,

1

though lasted for centuries, was grossly inaccurate. Additionally, in the Galenic view, blood was passed from the right side of the heart to the left side through pores, which was later shown to be incorrect as they do not exist within the inter-ventricular septum, as demonstrated by Columbus (1516-1559), a Belgian anatomist. Otherwise, this would be known as the septal defect. Columbus, during his many dissections, confirmed that venous blood of the right ventricle passed into the left ventricle through the lungs. This was concluded a few years earlier by Servetus (1511-1553), a Spanish theologian and physician. Thus, the open-circuit interpretation of the circulation by Galen cannot accurately describe the "circulation of blood".

In his many teachings, though some aspects were later known to be erroneous, Galen was nevertheless the first to recognize that the walls of arteries are thicker than those of the veins, and that arteries were connected to veins. It was the Persian physician Ibn al-Nafis (1210-1288) who claimed that venous blood of the right ventricle is carried by the artery-like vein into the lungs, where it mixes with the air and then into the left ventricle through vein-like artery.

Galileo Galilei (1564-1642) in his "Dialogue of the Two Sciences", which appeared in 1637, suggested the circulation of blood in a closed system. Centuries later today, the idea of the circulation of blood was credited to William Harvey (1578-1657), a contemporary of Galileo, in his now famous "De Motu Cordis and De Circulatione Sanguinis" (1628) presented to King Charles of England. He described in his "Anatomical Exercises" that "blood does continually passes through the heart" and that "blood flow continually out the arteries and into the veins". Harvey's work indicated the pulsatile nature of blood as a consequence of intermittent inflow, during roughly one-third of the heart cycle, now known as systole, in combination with essentially steady outflow through the periphery during the remaining cardiac period, the diastole.

Harvey's work was completed before Malphighi who worked with the aid of a compound microscope. He reported in 1661 the discovery of the capillaries linking the arterial circulation to the venous circulation, while he was working with the microscopic anatomy of the pulmonary parenchyma in the frog, an uni-ventricular amphibian. Dutch anatomist Van Leeuwenhoek (1632-1723) confirmed the capillaries in different organs of several animal species and established the concept of the capillary bed. Bypassing the capillaries are the arterio-venous anastomoses, which are now known to perform the function of controlling blood flow.

German anatomist Henle discovered the smooth muscle cells in small arteries in 1841. Thus, this provided the first evidence that smooth muscle contributes to arterial contraction. But it is not until almost a century later in 1937 that Zweifach showed that active contractility of the micro-vessels is confined to those vessels with smooth muscle cells.

In the investigation of the microcirculation, credit was given to Hall, an English physiologist, first to differentiate the capillaries from arterioles. The fact that capillaries transfer water and water-soluble substances from the blood stream to the surrounding tissues, were shown by Starling (1866-1927) and is now known as the Starling's hypothesis governing fluid exchange. The measurement of capillary blood pressure by cannulation was first performed in 1930, by Landis, in the nail microvascular bed (Mayrovitz, 1998). The ultra-structure of the microcirculation has now been established from electron microscope studies.

French physiologist Claude Bernard in 1852 showed that stimulation of sympathetic nerves induces vasoconstriction and the concept of controlling blood flow by vasomotor nerves. Neural control of the circulation is recognized as an important aspect in the regulation of vascular function.

Fascinated by anatomic structure of the vascular tree, as an art, Leonardo da Vinci (1452-1519) made many detailed drawings of the constituent parts of the circulatory system. He apparently already knew that both the contraction and resting periods are necessary for the heart to function with a normal rhythm. His anatomic drawings of the heart and the perfusing arteries are, to a large extent, amazingly accurate. This includes drawings of the heart and the great vessels, together with the main, anterior descending and circumflex coronary arteries and their major branches. Several drawings of the heart valves, demonstrating how well the leaflets are arranged when the valves are closed, as well as the detailed anatomic drawing of the neck arteries in man with its branching morphology were also shown (Li, 2000). In these, both the

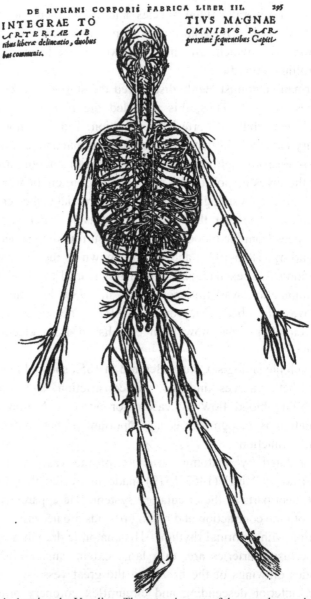

Fig. 1.1.1: Anatomic drawings by Vesalius. The extensiveness of the vascular tree is well appreciated.

length and angle of branching arteries are incredibly accurate. Vesalius (1514-1564), an anatomist, later provided a detailed drawing of the entire human vascular tree (Fig. 1.1.1).

Italian physician Caesalpinus apparently identified the pulmonary circulation and its associated two types of blood vessels: vena cava and pulmonary vein and pulmonary artery and aorta. Hooke (1635-1703; of Hooke's law of elasticity), an assistant of the English chemist Boyle (1627-1692; of Boyle's law of gases), recognized that respiration was necessary. But it was the English physiologist Lower (1631-1691) who continued the investigation to show the importance of ventilation-perfusion, i.e. exchange of gases between the lungs and blood. Gas transport in blood was reported by Magnus in 1837. He demonstrated that there was greater oxygen content in arterial blood and greater carbon dioxide content in the venous blood. Other formed elements, such as hemoglobin (Hb) were discovered by Funke in 1851 and has been shown as an important oxygen transporter. Neural effect was shown by Haldane (1860-1936), that carbon dioxide is a normal physiologic stimulus for the respiratory centers. The Haldane effect is now well appreciated in respiratory function and in oxygen therapy applications.

Lack of instrumentation, the measurements of the magnitudes of blood pressure and flow took considerably longer than the interpretation of the circulatory function. Hales in 1733 had incidentally already registered the magnitude of the blood pressure level about which blood oscillates. His initial measurement of blood pressure with a glass tube in a horse has been well illustrated in many publications. Thus, the magnitude of the mean arterial pressure and the amplitude of oscillation, or pulse pressure, were already known at that time. This forms the basis of modern day oscillometric measurement of blood pressure. Hales' measurements however, did not induce recognition of the great importance of blood pressure magnitude for many decades. We now know that significantly increased magnitudes of mean blood pressure and pulse pressure, the difference between systolic pressure and diastolic pressure, are major contributors to hypertension and many forms of cardiovascular diseases.

The shape of the pressure pulse became known only in the 19th century when Ludwig came up with the kymograph which inscribed blood pressure waveforms. His instrument provided information within a single beat which was a truly a technological advance at the time. Its accuracy was not comparable to present day instrument, although not an issue at the time. Blood pressure recording with the sphygmographs by Marey and his contemporary Mahomed has led to the clinical assessment of arterial diseases, such as hypertension. Incidentally, Chaveau and Marey (1863) also recorded cardiac chamber pressures. Both, shortly later, measured blood flow with an instrument they developed, now known as the bristle flowmeter.

Modern understanding of pressure-flow relationships came with the inventions of fluid-filled catheter-manometer system and the electromagnetic flowmeter. The simultaneous measurements of blood pressure and flow have led to considerable advancement of hemodynamics, or the studies of blood flow. The catheter was introduced in man by Forssmann in 1929, and later advanced for catheterization of the right heart for pressure measurement by Cournand and Range in 1941 (Li *et al.*, 1976). Cournand and Forssmann (together with Richards) shared the Nobel prize for medicine in 1956 for the invention leading to the advancement of modern day catheterization for visualization of blood pressure waveforms in various anatomical sites throughout the circulation. The electromagnetic flowmeter was introduced by Kolin in 1936. But ultrasonic transit-time and Doppler flow velocity probes have taken center stage in modern research and routine clinical measurements, mostly for their noninvasive monitoring capabilities.

In an attempt to understand the function of the arterial system as a whole, Hales (1733) concluded that in order for the arteries to accept the large amount of blood ejected, or the stroke volume, the arteries must behave like a temporary storage reservoir. Since the size of the aorta is considerably smaller than that of the ventricle, the receiving aorta must be elastic in order to perform the function as a reservoir. This interpretation of the reservoir function of arteries became known later as the Windkessel theory which was vigorously pursued a century later by a German physician Frank towards the end of the 19th century. The emphasis on the storage properties of the arteries modeled by Frank as a single elastic tube implied that all pressure fluctuations in the arterial tree should occur synchronously. In other words, the blood pressure pulse should propagate with infinite velocity. The peripheral vessels, on the other hand, are assumed rigid as stiff tubes. This gives rise to the lumped compliance-resistance model of the arterial circulation. This Windkessel model lacks the description of the propagation characteristics of the pressure pulse, but has remained the most popular model describing the arterial system and interpreting its physiological properties even until this day.

Blood pressure pulse propagation with finite wave velocity in a blood vessel was considered over two centuries ago by Euler in 1775. He attempted to develop a formula for its calculation. The well-known physicist Young in 1816, and also the Weber brothers in 1866, apparently solved for the propagation velocity in an elastic tube (Noordergraaf, 1969). Incorporating the elastic properties and geometry of the blood vessel, Moens (1878) and Korteweg (1878) separately developed what is now known as the Moens-Korteweg formula for the pulse wave velocity, or PWV:

$$c_0 = \sqrt{\frac{Eh}{2r\rho}} \tag{1.1.1}$$

where E is, appropriately at the time, defined as the Young's modulus of elasticity of the blood vessel, h and r are the wall thickness and inner radius of the uniform cylindrical vessel, respectively, and ρ is the density of blood. Pulse propagation velocity is seen to be related to the mechanical and geometrical properties of the blood vessel.

1.2 Importance of the Vascular System

In terms of the dynamics of the vascular system, the function of the heart is to provide energy and perfuse organ vascular beds. For the heart to accomplish this efficiently, the vascular system plays a central role as the distributing conduits. As such, both the distributing arteries and the peripheral vascular beds present the load to the pumping heart. Peripheral resistance has been popularly viewed in the clinical setting as the principal vascular load to the heart. This applies mainly to steady flow conditions. This description is naturally inadequate, because of the pulsatile nature of blood flow which remains throughout the microcirculation. Pulsatility implies that there is an oscillatory or pulsatile contribution to the vascular load to the heart. The significance of pulsations has been a popularly debated topic in the clinical settings where perfusion to organs is considered pertinent.

The vascular system provides a seamless illustration of an efficient transport system. This can be seen from the function of, for instances, the coronary circulation in perfusing the heart, the renal circulation in perfusing the kidneys, the cerebral circulation in perfusing the brain and the pulmonary circulation in perfusing the lungs. By virtue of the distributing arterial trees, oxygen, humoral agents, and nutrients be transported to the vital parts of the body, and at the same time, removal of biological waste materials is also accomplished.

1.3 Newer Concepts

Modern development of the theory related to blood flow in the vascular system has included multi-faceted aspects, such as, fluid mechanics, fluid-vessel interface, vascular tissue engineering, pulse wave trans-mission and mathematical modeling.

The mathematical formulations of blood flow through visoelastic arteries have been well established and documented in many texts (e.g. Noordergraaf, 1978, 2011; Li, 1987, 2000, 2004; Nichols and O'Rourke, 1998). These texts also provided experimental measurement methods and quantitative approaches to the assessments of the state of the arterial circulation. There are also several texts in describing the microcirculation and associated biomechanical behavior in greater detail (e.g. Lee and Skalak, 1989; Fung, 1997).

In the application to clinical situations, the interpretation of the morphology of blood pressure and flow waveforms in relation to underlying diseased conditions has attracted the most attention. The introduction of new groups of drugs beyond vasodilators, beta adrenergic blockers, calcium channel blockers and angiotensin-converting enzyme inhibitors that includes local targeted vascular drug delivery, as well as the introduction of gene therapy and regenerative medicine, to improve vascular perfusion and in the treatment of diseases, has become more avant garde.

Not only the arteries, the microcirculatory vessels are no longer viewed merely as resistance vessels, but are compliant with viscoelastic properties that vary with frequency. The classical elastic description of blood vessels has been modified to include viscosities of the blood and the vessel wall. The viscosities give rise to energy dissipation. Thus, the energy utilization and dissipation in relation to blood flow is now considered pertinent. Regarding Chi, or energy, the amount of the work that the heart has to generate during each beat has generated considerable attention. This included the steady energy dissipation through peripheral resistance vessels in different parts of the body, as well as energy required to overcome pulsations which persist even in the microcirculation.

Clinical applications of modern development of dynamics of the vascular system have initiated both invasive and noninvasive technological development and improvement in the accuracy of assessing the vascular structure and function. These include laser-Doppler velocimeter, multi-sensor pressure-velocity catheter, phase contrast magnetic resonance imaging (PC-MRI) and intravascular ultrasonic system (IVUS). There are also advancements in the development of interventional devices, such as local drug delivery catheter, laser- or balloon-angioplasty catheter, vascular stents and grafts. Many of these have been used for the assessment and treatment of vascular hypertrophy, stenosis and aneurysm, hypertension and atherosclerosis.

1.4 Book Contents

This book deals primarily with the dynamic behavior of the components of the vascular system and methods and techniques for their quantitative measurements. The book is written applying fundamental physical principles in conjunction with physiological measurements to the analysis of the structural and functional aspects of the vascular tree that includes the arterial circulation, the venous circulation, and the microcirculation, inclusive of arterioles, capillaries and venules. In addition, the constituent components, such as collagen, elastin, smooth muscle, and endothelial and red blood cells as well as transport phenomena are also discussed. An additional chapter on the interaction of the heart and the arterial system is also included in this second edition. Quantitative approaches are emphasized in the overall treatment.

In Chapter 2, modern concepts of vascular biology are illustrated. This begins with the anatomical organization of the vascular tree. Major branches of the aorta and some arteries at similar anatomic sites in some mammalian species, such as human, dog and rats, are described. These latter are common mammalian species where experimental measurements and data are most frequently collected. Geometric nonuniformities in terms of tapering and branching of the vessels are quantified. The fractal nature of the vascular tree can be well appreciated from some of the illustrations. The distributing channels and networking environment are illustrated.

Examination of structural properties allows us to differentiate the mechanical and functional characteristics of various vessels. This includes the nonuniformities in elasticity reflected in the content and organization of the walls of the various blood vessels. Constituent structural components of the arterial and venous wall are examined in rheological terms. In particular, the physical properties of elastin, collagen, and smooth muscle. The relative contents of the wall materials differentiate arteries from veins, arterioles and capillaries.

Oxygen is perhaps the most important component to be transported in the blood. The formed elements of blood are dealt with, that includes hemoglobin, red blood cells and plasma. Functional properties of blood are therefore included in this chapter. Some aspects of the circulating catacholamines and hormones, as well as neural control of the vascular system are equally important.

Chapter 3 deals with some fundamental concepts for analysis of the vascular system. The differences in their mechanical properties in large and small arteries and veins are examined. Their collective contributions to the overall function are analyzed. The arterial wall does not merely behave as an elastic vessel, therefore viscoelastic behavior becomes important. In this context, the viscous and elastic behavior of the composite, i.e. the arterial wall, is discussed. This includes the characteristics of a viscoelastic material, i.e. creep phenomenon, stress relaxation, and hysteresis. These aspects are also applied to veins, except the differences in distending pressures and collapsibility come into play.

Fundamental principles of fluid mechanics that includes classical laws and governing equations are provided. This includes Poiseuille's equation, Bernouilli's equation and the determining laminar and turbulent behavior in terms of Reynolds number. This is examined in terms of the rheology of blood flow to the containing vessel properties.

Engineering methods of basic analysis in the time domain, the Fourier analysis in the frequency domain are also included with examples that apply to the vascular system.

Chapter 4 deals with the hemodynamics of large arteries. Aorta is the largest artery whose distensibility and compliance facilitates ventricular ejection in systole. The pulsatile wave transmission characteristics of blood pressure and flow and simplified mathematical description, and fundamentals of modeling are included. The description classic of the windkessel model of the arterial system is first introduced. The windkessel is the mostly used lumped model and its analysis is elaborated in terms of total arterial system compliance and peripheral resistance. Extension of this model to more sophisticated later models include those that vary from a linear rigid tube model to a freely moving or constrained thin- or thick-walled, viscoelastic tube model. Some of these utilize Navier-Stokes equations describing fluid motion, Navier equations describing wall movement, and the equation of continuity describing the incompressibility of the blood. Experimental deviations from linear models are compared to nonlinear theories, so as to identify the regimes of nonlinearities.

Distributed model provide more precise descriptions of the pressure and flow behavior under varied conditions. However, they are generally complex and time-consuming in identify individual parameters, and less useful in daily clinical settings. Reduced models that are useful for practical and clinical applications are discussed. A recently introduced model to analyze the arterial wall behavior subject to varying pressure amplitudes in terms of pressure-dependent compliance is elaborated. This helps to explain the cyclical stress placed on the arterial wall and how the arterial wall adjust to rapidly changing pressure amplitudes.

Once models of the arterial system have been developed, it is necessary to verify the validity and limitations of these models. Such verifications depend often critically on the specific design of the experiments for measuring relevant hemodynamic parameters. For all practical purposes, these are pressure, flow, velocity, and vessel dimensions.

Pulsatile pressure and flow and their transmission characteristics are also the centerpoints of this chapter. Here, the peculiarities and features associated with pressure and flow waveforms measured in their respective anatomical sites are explained. How the vascular beds present as load to impede blood flow is quantitatively described in terms of the vascular impedance concept. Impedance, unlike resistance, which remains constant, is complex with its magnitude changes with frequency. Its usefulness is in its ability to include alterations in compliance, resistance and inertance. This provides a useful description of the changing arterial tree and individual vascular bed behavior. The manner by which pressure and flow pulses propagate and reflect can also be quantified.

Chapter 5 addresses the vascular branching aspects of the circulation, whether of arterial, venous or capillary, except the latter two are dealt in more detail in subsequent chapters. Branching geometry is examined in terms of morphological measurements. The basic fluid mechanic aspects of vascular branching in terms of pressure and flow transmission, shear stresses are explained, best with illustrations and mathematical formulations.

How efficient the pressure and flow pulses transmit depends on the propagation and reflection characteristics through different arteries and vascular branching junctions. Pulse wave velocity, a popularly used index to describe the vascular stiffness, is dependent on the geometric and elastic properties of the local arterial wall. Its measurement is therefore, elaborated.

With differing vascular impedances, wave reflections arise, because of the mismatching in impedances. The large peripheral resistances in the arterioles are the principal sites contributing to reflections. Increased wave reflection increases blood pressure amplitude and thus decreases flow. This reduces the pulse transmission efficiency for the propagating pulse. Pulse transmission through vascular branching junctions is dictated by the local blood vessel properties. For forward traveling wave, it is practically impedance-matched, resulting in optimal transmission. For the backward traveling wave towards the heart, it is greatly attenuated at the vascular branching. Thus, the design of the arterial tree is to facilitate pulse transmission to vascular beds. How this is optimized is explained.

Chapter 6 deals with the less studied aspects of the venous circulation, because of its low pressure and collapsibility and less life-threatening behavior. Blood volume is the highest at rest in the venous circulation, giving rise to its reservoir-like properties. The functional aspects of collapsibility and venous valves are also discussed, in terms of pressure-flow relations and the waterfall hypothesis. Modeling aspect is given in terms of mathematical descriptions and hydrodynamic set-ups.

Chapter 7 deals with the microcirculation. The greatest drop in mean blood pressure is found in the arterioles, hence justifying the vascular waterfall interpretation. How the contributions of the microcirculation to total peripheral resistance in its control of cardiac output are explained. The capillary circulation, for its vast networking and exchange environment is of utmost importance in terms of meeting the metabolic demand of the supplying tissues. The aspects of diffusion and cellular transports are of critical importance.

Thus, the design of the arterial tree is to facilitate pulse transmission to vascular beds. These latter are discussed in detail for their importance in both basic and clinical situations. Pulse pressure and flow remain pulsatile even in the microcirculation, albeit to a much more reduced amplitudes. The pulsatility facilitates capillary exchanges.

Chapter 8 deals with aspects of experimental methods, instrument-ation and devices that are widely used for hemodynamic measurements. Clinically useful methods and instruments for invasive and noninvasive determination of blood pressure flow, and vessel dimensions are first described. This begins with the commonly used noninvasive methods, such as auscultatory method, the sphygmomanometer cuff method and tonometry. Invasive blood pressure measurement system such as catheter-pressure transducer combination is also evaluated in terms of its frequency response.

Blood flow measurement with both electromagnetic flowmeter and Doppler ultrasonic method are described, as well as the technique of thermodilution measurement of cardiac output. The combination of

Doppler echocardiography and intravascular imaging devices now afford simultaneous flow velocity and lumen diameter measurements.

The final chapter, Chapter 9, on the interaction of the arterial system with the heart is a new addition to this second edition. Realizing that the arterial system is only perfused thorough its coupling with the heart, the aspect of the strength and timing of the cardiac contraction and its ejection are crucial in overall vascular function. The manner how ventricle and aorta interact will be explained, as well as the initial impulse aspect of ventricular ejection. Thus, the dynamics of the vascular system is only logically valid when the dynamics of the heart is included. While not making an attempt to address the entire regime of cardiac function, attempts are made to include the structural mechanical properties and the mechanisms of coupling of the heart to the arterial system, with particular emphasis on the left ventricle and the systemic arterial system. The current debate on the clinical observations of heart failure with preserved ejection fraction (HFpEF) and differentiating from those with reduced ejection fraction (HFrEF) are analyzed in terms of measurable hemodynamic parameters.

The aspect of cardiac assist device to aid the failing heart is well appreciated with the introduction of the intra-aortic balloon pump (IABP). IABP was selected because of the necessary consideration of the interaction of the left ventricle and the arterial system. Our experience with this in-series cardiac assist device is illustrated in terms of hemodynamic function. The dynamics of the assisted circulation is examined in terms of different modes of mechanical assistance.

The overall function of the dynamics of the vascular system depends not only on the anatomical structure of the individual vessels, but also on their multi-faceted functional interaction with neighboring and distant vessels, and, of course, with the heart. This will become apparent to the readers from the contents of this book.

Chapter 2

Vascular Biology, Structure and Function

2.1 Anatomical Organization of the Vasculature

2.1.1 *The Closed-loop Circulatory System*

The heart, the arterial systems, the venous systems and the micro-circulatory systems, coupled with neuro-humoral influences form the entire circulation. Each is an important functional complement that the circulatory system cannot be effectively described by its individual parts alone. By virtue of the distributing vascular trees, oxygen, humoral agents, and nutrients are transported to the vital parts of the body and the waste products are removed. The heart provides the necessary energy.

In terms of the general structure components, Fig. 2.1.1 suffices to provide an overview of the connectivity of the circulation.

2.1.2 *The Heart*

The heart in mammalian species has four chambers, the left ventricle (LV), the right ventricle (RV), left and right atria (LA and RA). The left ventricle pumps blood into the aorta through the aortic valve, perfuse the systemic arterial system and the right ventricle pumps blood into the main pulmonary trunk, perfuse the pulmonary arterial tree.

The shape of the left ventricle is in-between conical and semi-ellipsoidal with its narrow end forming the apex of the heart. These shapes, as well as cylinder and sphere, have been used in ventricular modeling and in image processing. The left ventricular wall is about three times as thick as the right ventricle, thus is able to develop a much higher pressure. The thick interventricular septum, separating the left and right ventricles, is more closely associated with the pumping action of the left ventricle. The ventricle also contracts much more in the short-axis (septum to LV free wall) or circumferential direction than the long-axis or base-to-apex direction. The ventricles are made up of muscular fibers. This so-called "myocardium" can be further divided transmurally into the inner endocardium and the outer epicardium.

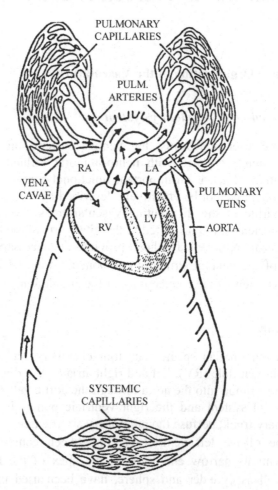

Fig. 2.1.1: Diagram illustrating the overall circulation. The four cardiac chambers (LV = left ventricle, LA = left atrium, RV = right ventricle, RA = right atrium) and systemic and pulmonary circulations are shown. Arrows indicate directions of blood flow.

There are four heart valves involved in the filling and pumping action of the heart. The mitral valve, with just two leaflets, situates between the left atrium and the left ventricle. It controls the flow between these two chambers, but is a one-way valve. The tricuspid valve, as the name implies, has three cusps. These are the posterior, the septal, and the anterior. The cusps have similar geometric shapes. The right ventricle and the low-pressure pulmonary arterial system on the other hand, are separated by the pulmonary valve. The aortic valve separates the left ventricle from the ascending aorta leading to the high pressure systemic arterial system. These valves have three leaflets and are of similar shape.

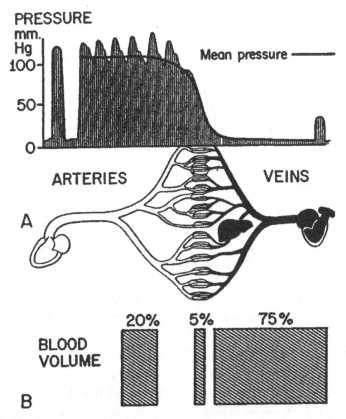

Fig. 2.1.2: Blood pressure and blood volume distribution of the systemic circulation. Notice the largest pressure drop occurs in the arterioles and the largest amount of blood volume reside in the veins which serve as reservoir. From Rushmer (1972).

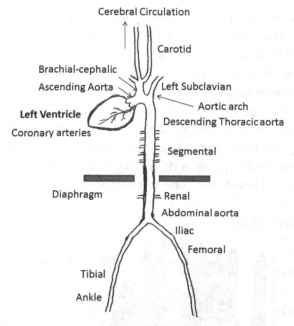

Fig. 2.1.3: Sketch of the mammalian arterial tree. Anatomic structures reveal branching characteristics of the arterial system.

2.1.3 *The Arteries*

Anatomical descriptions of the human and other mammalian vascular trees can be found in many textbooks. For the purpose of illustrating the blood perfusion and pressure pulse transmission path, the major branches of a typical mammalian arterial tree are shown in Fig. 2.1.3.

There are considerable similarities among the corresponding anatomical sites of the mammalian arterial circulation (Li, 1996). The root of the aorta begins immediately at the aortic valve. The outlet of the valve sits the ascending aorta having the largest diameter. The first branching off the aorta are the left and right main coronary arteries. The aortic arch junction is formed by the ascending aorta, the brachiocephalic artery, the left subclavian artery, and the descending thoracic aorta.

There are numerous branches come off the descending aorta at right angles, renal arteries which perfuse the kidneys are such examples. The distal end of the descending aorta is the abdominal aorta which forms the aorto-iliac junction with left and right iliac arteries and its continuation. In the human, it is a bifurcation. The femoral artery, a well-known peripheral artery, because of its accessibility, continues from the iliac artery. These are the arteries perfusing the upper thighs with the tibial arteries peruse the lower legs and leading to the ankle arteries. The aorta has, comparatively speaking, the greatest geometric taper, with its diameter decreasing with increasing distance away from the ventricle. The common carotid arteries are the longest, relatively uniform vessels, with the least geometrical tapering. The brachial arteries perfuse the upper arms leading to distal radial arteries. It is worth noting here that in humans, both brachial and radial arteries are the most common sites for noninvasive blood pressure monitoring, with radial in particular as wearable sensor site.

2.1.4 *The Veins*

Arteries deliver blood from the ventricles to vascular beds, while veins return it to the atria. Veins, unlike arteries are generally thin-walled and have low distending pressures. They are collapsible even under normal conditions of blood pressure pulsation.

The inferior vena cava is the main trunk vein. The superior vena cava feeds into the right atrium and the main pulmonary vein leads into the left atrium with oxygen enriched blood.

Veins have a greater total number than arteries and thus the venous system has a much larger cross-sectional area. This results in a much larger volume available for blood storage. Indeed, veins are known as low pressure storage reservoirs of blood. Under normal physiological conditions, the venous system contains about 75% of the total blood volume in the systemic circulation with the systemic arterial system constitutes some 15%. For this reason, veins are often referred to as capacitance vessels. Venous return is an important determinant of cardiac output. The pulmonary circulation contains about one quarter the blood volume of the systemic circulation.

Veins have much thinner walls and less elastin than arteries. Because of this, veins are stiffer than arteries. However, the low operating pressure and collapsibility allows veins to increase their volume by several times under a small increase of distending pressure.

There are bicuspid valves in veins. These valves permit unidirectional flow, thus preventing retrograde blood flow to tissues due to high hydrostatic pressures. These valves are notably present in the muscular lower limbs.

2.1.5 *The Microvasculature*

As stated previously, the function of the cardiovascular system is to provide a homeostatic environment for the cells of the organism. The exchange of the essential nutrients and gaseous materials occurs in the microcirculation at the level of the capillaries. These microvessels are of extreme importance for the maintenance of a balanced constant cellular environment. Capillaries and venules are known as exchange vessels where the interchange between the contents in these walls and the interstitial space occur across their walls.

The microcirculation can be described in terms of a network such as that shown in Fig. 7.1.1. It consists of an arteriole and its major branches, the metarterioles. The metarterioles lead to the true capillaries via a precapillary sphincter. The capillaries gather to form small venules, which in turn become the collecting venules. There can be vessels going directly from the metarterioles to the venules without supplying capillary beds. These vessels form arteriovenous (A-V) shunts and are called arteriovenous capillaries. The capillary and venule have very thin walls. The capillary, as mentioned before, lacks smooth muscle and only has a layer of endothelium. The smooth muscle and elastic tissue are present in greater amounts in vessels having vasoactive capabilities, such as arterioles. This is also the site of greatest drop in mean blood pressure. For this reason, arterioles are the principal contributors to peripheral vascular resistance that can effectively alter cardiac output.

The structural components of the microcirculation are classified into resistance, exchange, shunt, and capacitance vessels. The resistance vessels, comprising the arterioles, metarterioles, and precapillary sphincters, serve primarily to decrease the arterial pressure to the levels of the capillaries to facilitate effective exchange.

2.2 Geometric and Mechanical Properties of Blood Vessels

2.2.1 *Geometric Nonuniformity of Blood Vessels*

The arterial system is a tapered branching system. Changes in lumen size are often associated with branching and appropriate tapering. In the normal arterial system, the branched daughter vessels are always narrower than the mother vessel, but with slightly larger total cross-sectional areas. This means that the branching area ratio, or the ratio of the total cross-sectional area of the daughter vessels to that of the mother vessel, is slightly greater than one. This has significance in terms of pulsatile energy transmission.

Arterial diameters and lumen areas of the vascular tree can be determined from different imaging modalities, such as angiography, CT scan, ultrasound imaging or magnetic resonance imaging or from implanted sonomicrometers. Arteries in man and in dog retract some 25 to 40 percent when removed. It is therefore necessary that in-vivo lengths are restored and corresponding pressures are given for mechanical measurements. Under normal conditions, higher distending pressure leads to greater lumen diameter. Arterial vessel dimensions have been provided for the dog (McDonald, 1974) and man (Westerhof *et al.*, 1969). The latter were used for constructing the analog model of the human systemic arterial tree.

There are several branching junctions before the pulse reaches the vascular beds. In relation to this, the number of generations of blood vessels is of important consideration in terms of blood flow. These can be found in Green (1950) and Iberall (1967). Fractal studies of vascular tree structures utilize much of this information.

Experimental data give typical values of internal diameters in a 20 kg dog: ascending aorta, 15 mm; abdominal aorta, 8 mm; femoral artery, 3 mm; small artery, 0.1 mm. These values reveal an appreciable "geometric taper" in the aorta from the root to the aorto-iliac junction (Li, 1987). Together with branching, it contributes to the "geometric nonuniformity, observed throughout the arterial system. Corresponding data for the humans can be extrapolated with the use of allometry (Li, 1996; Li *et al.*, 2015).

The term "geometrical taper" is appropriate when applied to a single continuous conduit, such as the aorta. The area change of the aortic cross section is close to an exponential form and can be expressed as:

$$A(z) = A(0)e^{-kz/r} \qquad (2.2.1)$$

where:
z = distance in the longitudinal axial direction along the vessel
r = vessel lumen radius in cm
k = taper factor, dimensionless
$A(0)$ = the cross-sectional area at the entrance of the vessel in cm^2
$A(z)$ = the cross-sectional at distance z along the vessel in cm^2

The vessel area is calculated, assuming a circular cross-section,

$$A = \pi r^2 \qquad (2.2.2)$$

The taper factor k, can be readily obtained as

$$k = \frac{r}{z}\ln\frac{A(o)}{A(z)} \qquad (2.2.3)$$

Taper factor, *k*, for the aorta has been reported to be in the range of 0.0314-0.0367 for 20-30 Kg dogs (Li, 2000). Geometric taper factor can change substantially during varied vasoactive conditions and in disease conditions, such as atherosclerosis, stenosis or aneurysm. When vasoactive drugs are administered which have differential effects on large and small arteries, changes in taper factors from normal can be quite pronounced.

Alternative formula to calculate taper factor per unit length, or k_o, is expressed as follows:

$$A(z) = A(0)e^{-k_o z} \qquad (2.2.4)$$

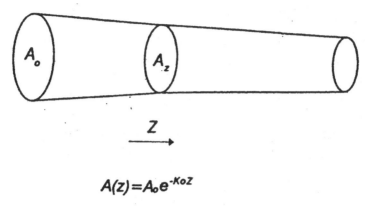

$$A(z) = A_o e^{-K_o z}$$

Fig. 2.2.1: Schematic diagram illustrating a blood vessel with geometric taper. The vessel diameter narrows with increasing distance (z) away from the origin. Geometric taper, an exponential function of distance, is normally calculated from the change in cross-sectional areas (A) as shown.

The reported values of k_o obtained for the abdominal aorta, the iliac, femoral and carotid arteries are shown in Table 2.2.1. These are measured in vivo at a mean arterial pressure of about 90 mmHg. The average body weights of dogs used are about 20 kg. It is obvious from these data that the taper factor is smaller for smaller vessels. Carotid arteries have the least taper. They are thus the best approximation to a geometrically uniform cylindrical vessel.

Area ratios calculated for vascular branching junctions were about 1.08 at the aortic arch, and 1.05 at the aorto-iliac junction (Li *et al.*, 1984). These values are slightly larger than 1.0. The hemodynamic consequences of these are discussed in Chapter 5.

Table 2.2.1: Measured external diameters and calculated taper factors in different arteries. Lower taper factor indicates more uniform longitudinal geometry.

	d (cm)	k_o (cm^{-1})
Abdominal aorta	0.777	0.027±0.007
Iliac artery	0.413	0.021±0.005
Femoral artery	0.342	0.018±0.007
Carotid artery	0.378	0.008±0.004

2.2.2 *Elastic Nonuniformity of the Blood Vessels*

In the broadest sense, the arterial wall (Fig. 2.2.2) consists of elastin, collagen, and smooth muscle embedded in a mucopolysaccharide ground substance. A cross section reveals the tunica intima, which is the innermost layer consisting of a thin layer (0.5-1 μm) of endothelial cells, connective tissue, and basement membrane. The next layer is the thick tunica media, separated from the intima by a prominent layer of elastic tissue, the internal lamina. The media contains elastin, smooth muscle, and collagen.

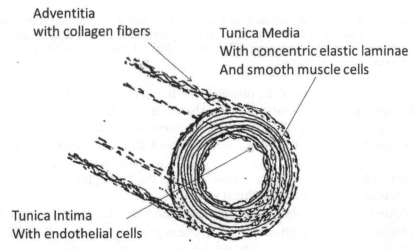

Fig. 2.2.2: Sketch of the cross sections of the artery reveal three distinctive layers: the innermost tunica intima, the thick tunica media, and the outermost adventitia.

The difference in their composition divides arteries into elastic and muscular vessels. The relative content of these in different vessels is shown in Fig. 2.2.3. All vessels, including the capillary, have endothelium. The capillary does not have smooth muscle content and has only a single layer of endothelial cells. The outermost layer is the adventitia which is made up mostly of stiff collagenous fibers.

Elastic laminae are concentrically distributed and attached by smooth muscle cells and connective tissue. Longitudinally, we find that the number of elastic laminae decreases with increasing distance from the aorta, but the amount of smooth muscle increases and the relative wall thickness increases. Thus, the wall thickness-to-radius ratio, or h/r is increased. The net stiffness is also increased, accounting for the increase in pulse wave velocity towards the periphery, as seen from the Moens-Korteweg formula. The mechanical behavior of peripheral vessels is largely influenced by the behavior of the smooth muscle, particularly by its degree of activation.

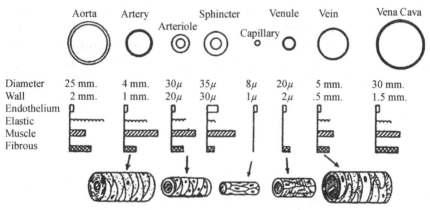

Fig. 2.2.3: Relative contents of endothelium, elastic and fibrous tissues, and smooth muscle in different vessels. Large arteries have more elastic and fibrous tissues whole smaller arteries have more smooth muscle in the tunica media. From Rushmer (1972).

2.2.3 *Vascular Stiffness and Elastic Properties*

Vascular stiffness is traditionally expressed in terms of Young's modulus of elasticity, which gives a simple description of the elasticity of the arterial wall. Young's modulus of elasticity (E) is defined by the ratio of tensile stress (σ_t) to tensile strain (ε_t). When the relationship between stress and strain is a linear one, then the material is said to be Hookian, or simply, it obeys Hooke's law of elasticity. This normally applies to a purely elastic material. It is only valid for application to a cylindrical blood vessel when the radial and longitudinal deformations are small compared to the respective lumen diameter or length of the arterial segment.

For the following analysis of the physical aspect of an artery, we shall consider a segment of the artery represented by a uniform isotropic cylinder with radius r, wall thickness h, and segment length *l*. Isotropy implies the uniform physical properties of the content of the arterial wall.

The arterial wall is actually anisotropic, consisting of various components discussed above, and the assumption of isotropy can not be exactly true. For instance, in vascular hypertrophy and in hypertension, selective thickening in tunica media is often observed. This can be accompanied by an increase in collagen and a decrease in elastin, and/or a change in the level of smooth muscle activation. These observed changes are not uniform throughout the arterial wall, i.e. anisotropic. Nevertheless, the isotropic assumption allows simpler quantitative descriptions of the mechanical behavior of the arterial wall properties and eases mathematical computation. The following formulae provide basic physical definitions.

Young's modulus of elasticity in terms of tensile stress and tensile strain is:

$$E = \frac{\sigma_t}{\varepsilon_t} \tag{2.2.5}$$

Stress has the dimension of pressure, or force (F) per unit area (A),

$$\sigma_t = \frac{F}{A} = P \tag{2.2.6}$$

where P is pressure, in mmHg or dynes/cm^2. Thus, stress has the dimension of mmHg or dynes/cm^2 in cm-g-sec or CGS units. The conversion of mmHg to dynes/cm^2 follows the formula that expresses the hydrostatic pressure above atmospheric pressure:

$$P = h \rho g \tag{2.2.7}$$

where h is the height in terms of the mercury column, ρ is the density of mercury, or 13.6 g/cm^3, and g is the gravitational acceleration. Hence 100 mmHg, or 10 cm Hg, is equivalent to

P = 100 mmHg = 10 x 13.6 x 980 = 133,280 dynes/cm^2 or about 1.33 10^5 dynes/cm^2. (2.2.8)

Of course, the choice in using N/m^2 or pascal is also common.

Strain in the longitudinal direction, or along the length of the blood vessel is expressed as the ratio of extension per unit length, or the ratio of the amount stretched longitudinally to the length of the original vessel segment,

$$\varepsilon_t = \frac{\Delta l}{l} \tag{2.2.9}$$

Strain in the radial direction, or perpendicular to the vessel segment length, is the fraction of distention of the vessel lumen radius or diameter. It is given by:

$$\varepsilon_r = \frac{\Delta r}{r} \tag{2.2.10}$$

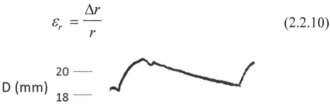

D (mm)

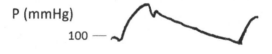

P (mmHg)

Fig. 2.2.4: Ultrasonic dimension gages recorded diameter of the aorta, together with aortic blood pressure. Calculation of radial strain can be obtained from the fractional change in diameter, $\Delta D/D$. This allows subsequent computation of pressure-strain elastic modulus, $Ep=\Delta P/(\Delta D/D)$, where ΔP is the pulse pressure.

As an example, the radial strain calculated from an ultrasonic dimension gage recording of the aortic diameter shown in Fig. 2.2.4 is

$$\varepsilon_r = \frac{1.93}{19.3} = 0.1 \tag{2.2.11}$$

In this case, the fractional change in diameter, or $\Delta D/D$, represents the radial strain.

Since pulsatile pressure and diameter tracings are rather similar (but with a distinct phase shift, i.e. pressure leads diameter or vice versa), many have utilized imaging modalities, such as ultrasound or magnetic resonance imaging of arterial lumen diameter changes to infer pressure changes. This has been done clinically for the noninvasive estimation of pulse wave velocity (PWV) – a pertinent index of vascular stiffness (Chapter 4).

For a blood vessel considered to be purely elastic, Hooke's law applies. To find the tension (T) exerted on the vessel wall due to intraluminal blood pressure distention, Laplace's law is useful. Laplace's law describes the tension exerted on a curved membrane with a radius of curvature. In the case of blood vessel, there are two radii of curvature, one that is infinite in the longitudinal direction along the blood vessel axis and the other is in the radial direction. Thus, Laplace's law for an artery can be written as:

$$T = p \cdot r \qquad (2.2.12)$$

This assumes the vessel has a thin wall or that the ratio of vessel wall thickness (h) to vessel lumen radius (r) is small, or $h/r \leq 1/10$. Here p is the intramural-extramural pressure difference, or the transmural pressure. When the vessel wall thickness is taken into account, the Lame equation becomes relevant:

$$\sigma_t = \frac{pr}{h} \qquad (2.2.13)$$

This relation is particularly importance in the analysis of aneurysm where increased lumen radius is accompanied by a decreased wall thickness, such that a further increase in distending pressure can cause rupture. In hypertension however, tension can be normalized by increasing the arterial wall thickness, chronically leading to observed vascular hypertrophy.

Arteries have been assumed to be incompressible. Although not exactly so, this is in general a good approximation. To assess the compressibility of a material, the Poisson ratio is defined. It is the ratio of radial strain to longitudinal strain. We obtain from the above definitions, the Poisson ratio as:

$$\sigma_n = \frac{\varepsilon_r}{\varepsilon_t} = \frac{\Delta r / r}{\Delta l / l} \qquad (2.2.14)$$

When radial strain is half that of longitudinal strain, or when $\sigma_n = 0.5$, the material is said to be incompressible. This means that when a cylindrical material is stretched, its volume remains unchanged. Or, in the case of an artery, when it is stretched, its lumen volume remains unchanged. Experimental measurements to obtain the Poisson ratio for arteries have shown σ_n to be close to 0.5. Arteries, therefore, can be considered to be close to being incompressible.

The above analysis assumes an isotropic arterial wall. The non-isotropy, or anisotropy, is seen in the various differences in the relative content and physical properties of the arterial wall. Collagen is the stiffest wall component, with an elastic modulus of 10^8 - 10^9 dynes/cm^2. This is some two orders of magnitude larger than those of elastin, 1-6 x 10^6 dynes/cm^2, and smooth muscle, 0.1-2.5 x 10^6 dynes/cm^2.

Elastin is relatively extensible, but is not a purely Hookean material. Collagen on the other hand is relatively inextensible, because of its high stiffness. Much more is known about vascular smooth muscle. Mechanical properties of arterial vessel walls can also be altered by neural mechanisms and by circulating catecholamine, such as norepinephrine. The composite of the arterial wall components operates in such a manner that at low pressures, elastin dominates the composite behavior. At high pressures, collagen becomes more important. Elastic modulus is a nonlinear function of pressure. The pressure dependence of the mechanical properties of arteries has been reported by several investigators (e.g. Cox, 1975; Weizsacker and Pascal, 1982; Drzewiecki *et al.*, 1997). Figure 2.2.5 illustrates how arterial lumen diameter, hence volume and compliance vary with changing transmural pressure. With increasing positive transmural pressure, arterial vessel diameter is distended (Weizsacker and Pascal, 1982), as expected, the corresponding compliance however, declines. With negative transmural pressure, the arterial area compliance decreases as the artery is under collapse. The decrease in compliance with increasing transmural pressure follows a negative exponential function.

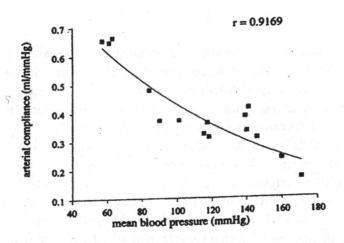

Fig. 2.2.5: Pressure dependence of mechanical properties of arteries is demonstrated in this figure. Compliance decreases with increasing pressure when the transmural pressure is positive and when the vessel is collapsing with negative transmural pressure.

Along the arterial tree, longitudinally, we find that the number of elastic laminae decreases with increasing distance from the aorta, but the amount of smooth muscle increases and the wall thickness-to-radius (h/r) ratio increases. The underlying vascular stiffness is thus increased. This latter phenomenon accounts for the observed large increase in pulse wave velocity (Chapter 4). The mechanical properties are largely influenced by the behavior of the smooth muscle. Its elastic properties and activation have attracted considerable interests. A longitudinal section also reveals a helical organization of the collagen fiber network. It is this network that contributes mostly to the anisotropic properties of the arterial wall.

2.3 Functional Properties of Blood

Blood is the principal vehicle and medium that serves to provide nutrients and remove waste products throughout the complex multi-cellular constituents of the body organs. It consists of a plasma fluid with a number of formed elements.

2.3.1 *Blood Plasma and Blood Gas*

Blood plasma is about 90-95% water and contains numerous dissolved materials that include proteins, lipids, carbohydrates, electrolytes, hormones and pigments. It is the proteins that dominant the characteristics of the plasma, which has a specific gravity (SG) of plasma, which is about 1.028. These are albumin, globulin and fibrinogen. The principal concentration by weight through fractionation electrophoresis shows that albumin which has the lowest molecular weight (69,000) exhibits the highest concentration of some 55%, followed by globulin (80,000-200,000) of about 38% and largest molecular weighted fibrinogen (350,000-400,000) of just 7%.

These proteins play an important functional role in viscosity, osmotic pressure and suspension characteristics of the plasma. Gases, such as oxygen and carbon dioxide are dissolved in the blood plasma. Their partial pressures can be derived from gas laws. We know that for an ideal gas, the pressure, volume and temperature are related by the gas law:

$$PV = nkT \qquad (2.3.1)$$

where P is the pressure, V is the volume, n is the number of gas molecules, k is Boltzmann's constant, and T is absolute temperature in Kelvin. The concentration, C_c, is normally expressed in terms of moles per unit volume,

$$C_c = \frac{n}{N_A V} \qquad (2.3.2)$$

where N_A is the Avogadro's number. Substitute for the universal gas constant $R = k N_A$ we have

$$P = C_c RT \qquad (2.3.3)$$

The partial pressure of a gas mixture, p_i, can be calculated knowing the molar fraction of the gas, f_i, and the total pressure, P, i.e.

$$p_i = f_i P \qquad (2.3.4)$$

When a gas with partial pressure p_i is in contact with a liquid, some of the gas will be dissolved in the liquid. Here we can define the solubility which is related to the concentration c_i of the gas, and its partial pressure:

$$S_i = \frac{c_i}{p_i} = \frac{n}{p_i V} \qquad (2.3.5)$$

Solubility in general is dependent on the total pressure above the liquid and temperature. Solubility of some gases in blood plasma is shown in Table 2.3.1.

Table 2.3.1: Solubility of gas in blood plasma.

Gas	Solubility in Molar/mmHg
O_2	1.4×10^{-6}
CO_2	3.3×10^{-5}
CO	1.2×10^{-6}
N_2	7.0×10^{-7}
He	4.8×10^{-7}

2.3.2 Oxygen Saturation Curves and Hemoglobin

The binding of oxygen with hemoglobin provides an efficient transport system to deliver and maintain a desirable amount of tissue and organ oxygenation. The oxygen saturation curve follows an S-shape as shown in Fig. 2.3.1. At a partial pressure of 100 mmHg, typical in the lungs and in arteries, hemoglobin is about 97% saturated. In veins and some tissues, the partial pressure of oxygen is about 40 mmHg. Here the saturation decreases to 75% or so. Since the slope of the curve changes greatly at this level, hemoglobin can easily give up its carrying oxygen readily when the metabolic need arises. This is accompanied by a drop in the partial pressure of oxygen, hence a reduced saturation of hemoglobin. Thus, the oxygen transport system is ideally designed to perform the tasks of on-demand metabolic adjustments. This is even better illustrated when oxygen is transferred from hemoglobin to myoglobin during greater muscle tissue demand. The affinity of myoglobin for oxygen is significantly greater than that of hemoglobin.

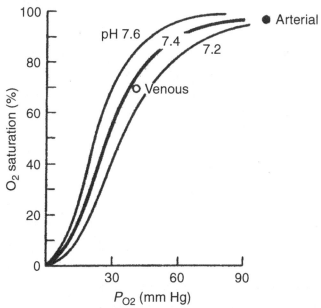

Fig. 2.3.1: Oxygen saturation curve displaying its S-shaped characteristics. Normal arterial and venous blood O_2 saturations are also indicated. Normal arterial O_2 saturation is about 96%.

The oxygen affinity decreases with decreasing pH. This is termed the Bohr effect by which changes in blood PCO_2 which affects blood pH, indirectly also influence hemoglobin-oxygen affinity.

Hemoglobin consists of four polypeptide chains or globins and four disc-shaped molecular ring or *heme* groups, allowing binding of four oxygen molecules. Once bound with oxygen, the iron atoms in hemoglobin give it the red color. Optical absorptions of hemoglobin and oxy-hemoglobin (Fig. 2.3.2) can be readily monitored by near-infrared spectroscopy. The isobestic point, when the two absorptions are equal which can be used as a reference, is at 805 nm.

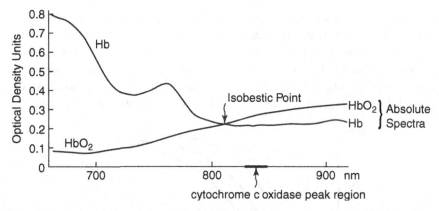

Fig. 2.3.2: Optical absorptions of hemoglobin (Hb) and oxy-hemoglobin (HbO₂). The isobestic point where the absorptions are equal is at about 805 nm. Cytochrome c oxidase absorption region is also indicated.

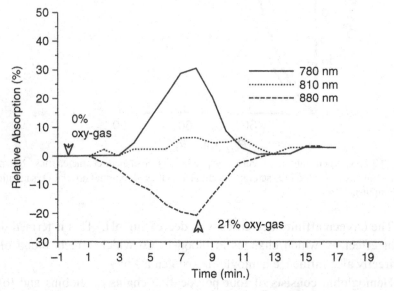

Figure 2.3.3: Relative absorption response of the near-infrared oxygenation monitoring during cerebral hypoxia, induced via reduced O₂ supply (arrow) and return to normal 21% oxygen-gas mixture (arrow). 810 nm is used to track the reference isobestic point when the absorptions are equal, while 880 nm and 780 nm track oxygenated and deoxygenated hemoglobin, respectively.

Figure 2.3.3 demonstrates the rapid changes in brain oxygenation, for instance, due to hypoxia (Li *et al.*, 2010). During the experiments, the fraction of normal inspired oxygen or FiO_2 of 21% was replaced with 100% N_2 gas via the respirator for seven minutes, the maximal tolerable limit. The gas supply is subsequently changed to FiO_2 of 50% or 21% O_2 at room air to alter oxygenation level. Absorptions were measured at 780 nm (for detection of Hb concentration), 810 nm (isobestic reference) and 880 nm (for detection of concentration of HbO_2), by applying light emitters and detectors noninvasively over the frontal skull. It is seen that oxygenated hemoglobin declines rapidly beginning at the onset of hypoxia, while deoxygenated hemoglobin correspondingly and rapidly increased. The total blood volume, as indicated by the isobestic reference remains largely unchanged.

2.3.3 *Red Blood Cells, Hematocrit and Blood Volume*

The principal formed elements are erythrocytes or red blood cells (RBC or rbc), leukocytes or white blood cells and thrombocytes.

The principal function of the red blood cell is in the transport of oxygen (O_2) and carbon dioxide (CO_2). The concentration of hydrogen ion (pH) determines the acidity/alkalinity. These three quantities (pO_2, pCO_2 and pH) are the principal components involved in the blood gas analysis. Some of the definitions from blood sample analysis are shown below:

$$pH = \frac{1}{\log[H^+]} \tag{2.3.6}$$

$$Hematocrit, or Hct(\%) = \frac{Re\, dBloodCells}{Blood} \times 100 \tag{2.3.7}$$

$$Fcr = \frac{Hct(totalbody)}{Hct(venous)} \tag{2.3.8}$$

Mean corpuscular volume is defined as

$$MCV = \frac{HematocritRatio \times 10^3}{RBCcount(10^6 / mm^3)} \qquad (2.3.9)$$

Mean corpuscular hemoglobin is defined as

$$MCH = \frac{Hemoglobin(g/L)}{RBCcount(10^6 / mm^3)} \qquad (2.3.10)$$

Blood volume is normally determined by the sum of the red blood cell volume (V_{rbc}) and the plasma volume (V_p):

$$V_B = V_{rbc} + V_p \qquad (2.3.11)$$

The total blood volume in a normal 70 Kg adult is about 5 liters. This value is not constant and changes according to properties of the vascular system and activity.

Although total blood volume (TBV) can be obtained from dilution techniques, an estimate of the total blood volume can be obtained from a single determination of red blood cell volume or plasma volume and corrected venous hematocrit from the following expressions:

$$BV = \frac{V_p}{(100 - Hct) \times Fcr} \qquad (2.3.12)$$

$$BV = \frac{V_{rbc}}{Hct \times Fcr} \qquad (2.3.13)$$

Indicator dilution techniques are commonly employed in the determination of blood volume. For instance, for the determination of plasma volume, small amount (5 microcurie) of radioactively iodinated (I^{125}) serum albumin (RISA) is injected into the circulation and its concentration sampled. For determination of red blood cell volume, radioactive labeling (e.g. chromium ^{51}Cr) of red blood cells have been used and again, concentration of injected sample determined for a prescribed intervals.

Table 2.3.2: Diameters of red blood cells (RBC) of some mammalian species.

Species	Body weight (kg)	RBC Diameter (μm)
Shrew	.01	7.5
Mouse	.20	6.6
Rat	.50	6.8
Dog	20	7.1
Man	70	7.5
Cattle	300	5.9
Horse	400	5.5
Elephant	2000	9.2

Data from Altman and Dittmer (1961) have shown that in more than one hundred mammalian species, the "red blood cells" are of similar size. If we compare the size of red cells from various mammals, we find the perhaps surprising fact that their diameters seem to be rather uniform and independent of mammalian body size (Table 2.3.2).

2.4 Control Aspects of the Vascular System

Homeostasis and overall control of the circulation hinge on the regulation and control of blood pressure and maintaining adequate perfusion to vital organ vascular beds. In addition, the delivery of oxygen and nutrients and the removal of carbon dioxide and metabolic waste products are also important considerations. Controlling blood pressure is necessary to ensure adequate and on-demand supply of blood to the heart and the brain and, also, to the rest of the body organs. Control of capillary pressure is necessary to maintain tissue volume and the composition of the interstitial fluid within desirable ranges.

Various receptors of the body are anatomically structured to sense and monitor the state of the heart and the vascular system. In response to sensory inputs from these receptors, either individually or in an integrated manner, both neural and chemical signals induce adjustments to maintain arterial pressure, blood flow and other hemodynamic variables.

2.4.1 *Control of the Central Cardiovascular System*

Arterial baroreceptors sense and monitor blood pressure at various sites in the cardiovascular system. They are principally located at the aortic arch and the carotid sinus. Responses from these baroreceptors, together with those of chemoreceptors are transmitted to the brain. The chemoreceptors which monitor the CO_2, O_2, and pH of the blood are located principally at the aortic body and the carotid body.

There are also mechanoreceptors in the heart (i.e. atrial mechanoreceptive afferent fibers), as well as thermoregulatory receptors, that initiate appropriate reflex effects on the overall cardiovascular system. Additionally, skeletal muscle contraction or changes in the composition of the extracellular fluid of tissues can activate afferent fibers which are embedded in the muscle or tissue to cause changes in the cardiovascular system.

Sensory inputs are temporally and spatially integrated at regions that contain neurons in the brain occupying space known as the cardiovascular center. This region is located at the medulla oblongata and pons. The medullary cardiovascular center also receives inputs from other regions of the brain, including the medullary respiratory center, hypothalamus, and cerebral cortex. The output from the medullary cardiovascular center feeds into sympathetic and parasympathetic autonomic motor neurons that innervate the heart and the smooth muscle of arterioles and veins, as well as to other brain neurons.

The autonomic nervous system consists of two principal trunks: the sympathetic nervous system and the parasympathetic system. Stimulation of sympathetic nerves increases the rate and force of contraction of the heart and causes vasoconstriction which increases arterial blood pressure. The stimulation of parasympathetic nerves, cause a decrease in arterial blood pressure. The opposing effects of these two systems on blood pressure are sensed by two functionally different regions of the medullary cardiovascular center. These are known as the pressor and depressor regions. Stimulation of the pressor center results in sympathetic activation and an increase in blood pressure. Stimulation of the depressor center results in parasympathetic activation and a decrease in blood pressure.

2.4.2 *Functions of the Baroreceptors*

Baroreceptors are located in the carotid sinus and the aortic arch. There are two types of baroreceptors. The unmyelinated baroreceptors are localized in the central cardiovascular system and respond to pressures above normal and initiate reflexes to reduce arterial blood pressure. The myelinated baroreceptors respond to blood pressures below normal and thus protecting the cardiovascular system from prolonged reduction in blood pressure. The carotid sinus and aortic arch perform similar functions and differ only slightly in terms of structure.

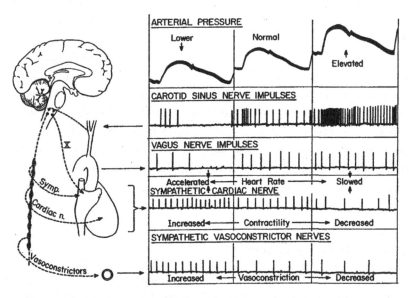

Fig. 2.4.1: Discharge frequencies of carotid sinus stretch receptors in the control of blood pressure, via sympathetic and vagal stimulations. From Rushmer (1972).

A perturbation that gives rise to an increase in blood pressure stretches the wall of the carotid sinus. This in turn causes an increase in discharge frequency from the baroreceptors (Fig. 2.4.1). When the pressure is low, the pressor-receptor impulse frequency decreases, the vagus nerve impulses diminish and sympathetic cardiac nerve impulses increase to accelerate the heart rate. This is accompanied by increased activation of sympathetic vasoconstrictor fibers. The result is an increase in peripheral resistance, hence an increase in blood pressure towards normal level. With an increase in blood pressure the carotid sinus impulse frequency decreases, reducing the sympathetic discharge and increasing the vagal discharge. The accompanied slowing in heart rate and peripheral vasodilation restores blood pressure to normal level.

A sigmoidal relationship between blood pressure and baroreceptor impulse frequency has been found and the system is most sensitive over the physiological range of blood pressures. It has been shown that the baroreceptor discharge frequency is higher when pressure is pulsatile than when it is steady and that the carotid sinus baroreceptors are most sensitive to frequencies of pressure oscillation between 1 and 10 Hz.

An increase in blood pressure sensed by baroreceptors is signaled to the medullary cardiovascular center, which in turn, through autonomic motor neurons, initiates a reflex reduction in both cardiac output and peripheral vascular resistance. The reduction in cardiac output results from both a decreased heart rate and a reduced force of cardiac contraction results in a decrease in arterial blood pressure. Thus the baroreceptor reflex of the carotid sinus is a negative feedback loop that tends to stabilize arterial blood pressure at a particular set point. This set point concept has been instrumental in understanding many physiological control mechanisms.

2.4.3 *Arterial Chemoreceptors*

Chemoreceptors are located in the carotid and aortic bodies. These chemoreceptors respond with an increase in discharge frequency to an increase in CO_2 or to decreases in O_2 and reduced pH of the blood perfusing the carotid and aortic bodies. Because CO_2 and O_2 are intimately related to the ventilation-perfusion process, chemoreceptors are particularly important in regulating ventilation.

An increase in discharge frequency of the chemoreceptor results in peripheral vasoconstriction and a slowing of the heart rate.

Vasoconstriction can result in an increase in blood pressure, which in turn can stimulate the baroreceptor to cause a reflex decrease in blood pressure. Thus, chemoreceptors have a direct effect on heart rate and an indirect effect on blood pressure.

Smooth muscle can exert influence on large vessels such as the aorta. Its activity in smaller arteries is greater, because of the increased wall thickness-to-radius ratio. With varied vasoactivity, arterial lumen can be modulated to regulate perfusion. Considerable variations in the constituent wall components, collagen, elastin and smooth muscle can be observed. Geometric change, such as the increased wall thickness-to-radius ratio is clearly visible.

Chapter 3

Physical Concepts and Basic Fluid Mechanics

3.1 Basic Mechanics and Dimensional Analysis

3.1.1 *Mass, Length and Time System and the Pi-theorem of Buckingham*

Description of physical quantities requires the use of dimensions. The mass (M), length (L) and time (T) representation of a physical variable or parameter, or the so-called the MLT system is the most common. Dimensional analysis has its well-founded place in the physical sciences and engineering.

We must differentiate between physical quantities and physical constants. The former always possess units, while the latter are not always dimensionless (e.g. Planck's constant). The use of Buckingham's Pi-theorem for dimensional analysis requires all physical quantities be expressed in M (mass), L (length) and T (time). The theorem has wide applications, as will be shown later.

Dimensional homogeneity, another requirement in order to use the Pi-theorem, was first proposed by Fourier in 1882, who stated that any equation applied to physical phenomena or involving physical measurements must be dimensionally homogeneous. Its usefulness can be found in the Navier-Stokes equations describing incompressible fluid flow in the longitudinal direction, in a blood vessel, for instance, (in cylindrical coordinates). Every term in the equation has the dimension of a pressure gradient for flow in the z direction: dp/dz, i.e. $M^1L^{-1}T^{-2}/L$ or $M^1L^{-2}T^{-2}$.

Many dimensionless numbers have found their way through the use of the dimensional matrix. The matrix comprises columns representing

43

physical quantities, while rows are filled with basic units (M, L, T). To form a dimensional matrix, a priori knowledge of pertinent physical parameters is necessary. For instance, if 8 physical quantities are important for the description of blood flow in arteries, and there are 3 basic units (M, L, T) to represent them, then we are be able to obtain 8-3=5 dimensionless pi-numbers. In general, the number of dimensionless pi-numbers are determined by the number of physical quantities minus the rank of the dimensional matrix.

To use the MLT system, one needs to first express explicitly any variable in its physical units, either using the CGS (cm, g, s) or the MKS (m, Kg, s) system or SI units of representation. For instance, blood pressure is commonly measured in mmHg and must be converted to g/cm s^2. Thus, pressure (p) is given as force (F) per unit area (A),

$$p = \frac{F}{A} = [M][L]^{-1}[T]^{-2} \qquad (3.1.1)$$

where A has the dimension of cm^2, or $[L]^2$, and force is mass times acceleration, Newton's second law,

$$F = m \cdot a = [M][L]/[T]^2 \qquad (3.1.2)$$

where a is the acceleration in cm per sec per sec, or cm/s^2 ($[L]/[T]^2$).

The left ventricular volume V, has the unit of ml or cm^3, and a dimension of

$$V = [L]^3 \qquad (3.1.3)$$

The aortic flow Q, represented by the rate of change of ventricular volume, has the unit of ml/s, or

$$Q = \frac{dV}{dt} = [L]^3 /[T] \qquad (3.1.4)$$

Linear flow velocity has the dimension of

$$v = \frac{dz}{dt} = [L]/[T] \tag{3.1.5}$$

or with a physical unit of cm/sec; z is along the axis of the direction of blood flow.

Heart rate in beats per minute or per second has the dimension of

$$f_h = [T]^{-1} \tag{3.1.6}$$

3.1.2 *Dimensional Matrix*

When formulating a dimensional matrix, it is necessary to identify the parameters that are considered pertinent to the problem at hand. These parameters need to be expressed in terms of [M] [L] and [T]. For example, given arterial blood pressure (p), flow (Q) and heart rate (f_h), a dimensional matrix can be formed

$$
\begin{array}{c c c c}
 & p & Q & f_h \\
M & 1 & 0 & 0 \\
L & -1 & 3 & 0 \\
T & -2 & -1 & -1
\end{array}
\tag{3.1.7}
$$

This is therefore, a 3 x 3 matrix, or a square matrix.

As another example, suppose that one wishes to examine the relationship between left ventricular wall tension (T) and left ventricular diameter or radius (r) and left ventricular pressure (knowingly, this is the Laplace's law), then a dimensional matrix can be formed in terms of the three parameters, prior to the application of Buckingham's Pi-theorem. This dimensional matrix is:

$$
\begin{array}{c c c c}
 & T & p & r \\
M & 1 & 1 & 0 \\
L & 0 & -1 & 1 \\
T & -2 & -2 & 0
\end{array}
\tag{3.1.8}
$$

Again, this is a 3 x 3 square matrix.

3.1.3 *Biological Scaling and Dynamics Similitude in Vascular Biology*

Dimensionless numbers provide useful scaling laws, particularly in multi-scale modeling and similarity transformation. Dimensional analysis is a powerful tool, not limited to just mathematics, physics and modeling, but has immense applicability to many biological phenomena (Li, 2000).

Despite its many useful applications, dimensional analysis is not without shortfalls. For a given set of physical quantities and basic units, we can generate new dimensionless numbers, which are not necessarily always invariant for a given system. They cannot therefore, be regarded as similarity criteria. The definition of dimensionless numbers as similarity criteria (Stahl, 1963), is therefore inadequate.

Let us consider blood flow in vessels and see how similarity criteria are obtained. A dimensional matrix is first formed by incorporating parameters that are pertinent to the analysis. These are the fluid density (ρ) and viscosity (η), diameter (D) of the blood vessel, velocities of the flowing blood (v) and of the pulse wave (c). In terms of the dimensioning mass (M), length (L) and time (T) system, we can write down the following dimensional matrix,

	ρ	c	D	η	v
	(g/cm^3)	(cm/s)	(cm)	(poise)	(cm/s)
M	1	0	0	1	0
L	-3	1	1	-1	1
T	0	-1	0	-1	-1
	k_1	k_2	k_3	k_4	k_5

$$(3.1.9)$$

where k_n's are Rayleigh indices referring to the exponents of the parameters. According to Buckingham's Pi-theorem (Li, 1983, 1986), two dimensionless pi-numbers (5-3 = 2) can be deduced.

Mathematically, we have

$$\pi_i = \rho^{k1}\ c^{k2}\ D^{k3}\ \eta^{k4}\ v^{k5} \tag{3.1.10}$$

or in terms of M, L and T, then

$$\pi_i = (M^{k1}L^{-3k1}T^0)\ (M^0L^{k2}T^{-k2})\ (M^0L^{k3}T^0)$$
$$(M^0M^{k4}L^{-k4}T^{-k4})\ (L^{k5}T^{-k5}) \tag{3.1.11}$$

Since pi-numbers are dimensionless, this means the exponent needs to be zero. Equating the exponents of M, L and T to zero and solve, we obtain two pi numbers or similarity criteria (Li, 1983):

$$\pi_1 = \frac{\rho v D}{\eta} = \mathrm{Re} \qquad \text{and} \qquad \pi_2 = \frac{c}{v} = \frac{1}{Ma} \tag{3.1.12}$$

The first pi-number is clearly identified as the Reynolds number, Re. The second is the inverse of the Mach number, *Ma*. The Mach number in terms of sound velocity is the ratio of flow speed to the local sonic speed, or in this case the ratio of flow velocity to the pulse wave velocity in terms of blood pulse wave propagation. It is also termed the velocity fluctuation ratio (VFR). Recalling that to assume linearity of the arterial system, the flow velocity should be small as compared to the pulse wave velocity, or that VFR should be small.

The requirements for dynamic similarity (Rosen, 1978) are that two flows must possess both geometric and kinematic similarity. Thus the effects of, for instance, viscous forces, pressure forces, surface tension, (Li, 1996) need to be considered. Here we have only the ratio of inertial forces to viscous forces i.e. Reynolds number, and the ratio of inertial forces to compressibility forces i.e. Mach's number or velocity fluctuation ratio. For a truly incompressible fluid, c>>v such that Ma = 0. For the analysis of blood flow in arteries, both blood and arterial walls are normally assumed to be incompressible. The Poisson ratio (σ_p), which is the ratio of radial strain to longitudinal strain (eqn. 3.1.20), for the aorta is about 0.48, close to an incompressible material (σ_p=0.5). As mentioned above, the assumptions of linearity and linear system analysis applied to hemodynamic studies often require the ratio v/c<<1 (flow velocity to pulse wave velocity), or that the diameter of the blood vessel is small as compared to the pulse propagation wavelength, D/λ<<1. This is justified during the large part of the cardiac cycle. At peak flow rates in early systole however, the ratio of v/c is large (but not exceeding 1), turbulence may ensue to produce nonlinear effects.

Reynolds number from eqn. (3.1.12) is seen to vary with body length dimensions, or the diameter of the aorta. One question immediately arises is that the resulting Reynolds numbers calculated for large mammals, such as the horse, show that turbulence may occur for a large portion of the systole in the aorta. But this may not necessarily be the case. It has been well documented that turbulence may not exist even for Reynolds number greatly exceeding the critical value of 2,000. It is only established that for Reynolds number under 2,000, turbulence does not normally occur. Again, this value was established under steady flow conditions in rigid tubes. This differs from pulsatile flow in elastic arteries.

The arterial blood flow exhibits pulsatile characteristics and peripheral outflow occurs mostly in diastole. In systole during ventricular ejection, the aorta distends as a reservoir to accommodate the flow as described by the classic Windkessel model of the arterial system (Chapter 4). In concert with the pulsation, this compliance of the aorta acts to protect the peripheral vascular beds from sudden surges in pressure and flow. The compliance, defined as the ratio of change in volume due to a change in pressure,

$$C = dV/dP \qquad\qquad (3.1.13)$$

is proportional to body weight. A larger volume change occurs in the aorta of a larger mammal and the longer effective length of the aorta and a much slower heart rate, all help to reduce the tendency of turbulence to reside in too large a portion of systole.

3.1.4 *Elastic and Viscoelastic Properties of Blood Vessels*

Many investigators have examined elastic properties of arteries. It is found that the stress-strain or length-tension relationship is nonlinear and thus does not obey Hooke's law. Arterial elasticity increases with extension and the length-tension relation is curvilinear. Many experiments, however, were done in-vitro situations, having the advantage of well-controlled experimental conditions, but the disadvantage of extending the results to equate with in-vivo parametric changes.

A material that obeys Young's modulus of elasticity in terms of tensile stress and tensile strain is:

$$E = \frac{\sigma_t}{\varepsilon_t} \tag{3.1.14}$$

Stress has the dimension of pressure (p), or force (F) per unit area (A),

$$\sigma_t = \frac{F}{A} = p \tag{3.1.15}$$

where P is pressure, in mmHg or dynes/cm^2. Thus, stress has the similar dimension of mmHg or dynes/cm^2 in cm-g-sec or CGS units.

Strain in the longitudinal direction, or along the length of the blood vessel is expressed as the ratio of extension per unit length, or the ratio of the amount stretched longitudinally to the length of the original vessel segment,

$$\varepsilon_t = \frac{\Delta l}{l} \tag{3.1.16}$$

Strain in the radial direction, or perpendicular to the vessel segment length, is the fraction of distention of the vessel lumen radius or diameter. It is given by

$$\varepsilon_r = \frac{\Delta r}{r} \tag{3.1.17}$$

For a blood vessel considered to be purely elastic, Hooke's law applies. To find the tension (T) exerted on the arterial wall due to intra-luminal blood pressure distention, Laplace's law is useful. Laplace's law describes the tension exerted on a curved membrane with a radius of curvature. In the case of blood vessel, there are two radii of curvature, one that is infinite in the longitudinal direction along the blood vessel axis and the other is in the radial direction. Thus, Laplace's law for an artery can be written as:

$$T = p \cdot r \tag{3.1.18}$$

This assumes the artery has a thin-wall or that the ratio of arterial wall thickness (h) to arterial lumen radius (r) is small, or $h/r \leq 1/10$. Here p is the intramural-extramural pressure difference, or the transmural pressure. When the arterial wall thickness is taken into account, the Lame equation becomes relevant:

$$\sigma_t = \frac{pr}{h} \tag{3.1.19}$$

Arteries have been assumed to be incompressible. Although not exactly so, this is in general a good approximation. To assess the compressibility of a material, the Poisson ratio is defined. It is the ratio of radial strain to longitudinal strain. We obtain from the above definitions, the Poisson ratio as:

$$\sigma_n = \frac{\varepsilon_r}{\varepsilon_t} = \frac{\Delta r / r}{\Delta l / l} \tag{3.1.20}$$

When radial strain is half that of longitudinal strain, or when $\sigma_n = 0.5$, the material is said to be incompressible. This means that when a cylindrical material is stretched, its volume remains unchanged. Or, in the case of an artery, when it is stretched, its lumen volume remains unchanged. Experimental measurements to obtain the Poisson ratio for arteries have shown σ_n to be about 0.48, or close to 0.5. Arteries, therefore, can be considered to be close to being incompressible.

A purely elastic material differs from a viscoelastic material. The former depends only on strain (eqns. 3.1.16 and 3.1.17) while the latter depends on the rate of change of strain, or strain rate ($d\varepsilon/dt$) also. The artery as a viscoelastic material exhibits stress-relaxation, creep, and hysteresis phenomena (Fig. 3.1.1).

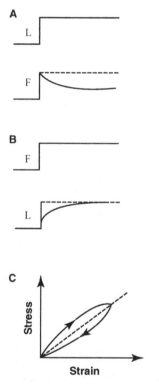

Fig. 3.1.1: Diagram illustrating the characteristics of a viscoelastic biological material such as the arterial wall: (A) stress relaxation: a step increase in length, L, or diameter results in an increase in force or tension which declines over time (x-axis) to a lower level, (B) creep phenomenon: with a step increment in applied force, the arterial length or diameter increases, but gradually and (C) hysteresis; with increase in stress, strain increases, but when the stress is removed, the strain follows a different path, resulting in a "hysteresis loop" indicating energy loss.

If a strip of artery is subjected to a step change in length, it will result in an initial increase in stress, and then decays to a lower value. This is known as stress-relaxation. There is a finite amount of time the vessel takes to relax. This is described by a time constant, which differs in different arteries. When an artery is subjected to a stepwise change in stress, its length will gradually increase to a constant value. This is the so-called, "creep phenomenon". As with stress relaxation, the increase in length or diameter, also takes a finite amount of time and is also subscribed to a time constant. These properties allow arteries to respond to rapid transient changes in transmural blood pressures.

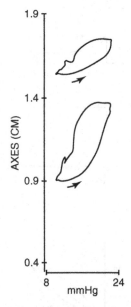

Fig. 3.1.2: Pressure-diameter relation of the main pulmonary artery showing hysteresis loops. Top tracing: major axis. Bottom tracing: minor axis. The difference in hysteresis loops is due to the non-cylindrical oval cross-sectional shape of the main pulmonary artery.

Hysteresis develops when the vessel is subjected to sinusoidal or cyclic changes. If the artery is purely elastic, there will be no phase shift between the applied pressure and the resulting change in diameter. The viscoelastic behavior of the artery leads to phase shifts in its pressure-diameter relation. A hysteresis loop is observed, reflecting viscous losses. In other words, energy is dissipated in stretching the artery and allowing it to return to its control value. If the artery were purely elastic, there would be no energy loss and the artery would return to its control value along the exact path during stretching.

Examples of experimentally measured pressure-diameter relations are shown in Fig. 3.1.2 for the pulmonary aorta. Since the pulmonary aorta is normally oval, there are two different diameters, namely, the major axis diameter and the minor axis diameter. When the major and minor axes diameters are plotted against pressure, the hysteresis loops are clearly seen. It is also clear that the pulmonary aorta is stiffer (less diameter distention with increasing pressure) along the major axis than the minor axis. In small peripheral vessels the viscous modulus is larger and the phase shift becomes more pronounced. This can be seen in the simultaneously measured pressure-diameter relation obtained for the femoral artery, for instance.

The static modulus of elasticity differs from the dynamic elastic value. Measurement of dynamic elasticity has gained considerable attention, mainly because of its applicability to pulsatile conditions. The approach employs the measurement of pressure-diameter relations, and the subsequent calculations of the incremental elastic modulus (E_{inc}) which is complex (E_c):

$$E_{inc} = E_{dyn} + \eta\omega \qquad (3.1.21)$$

When an elastic modulus is complex, it implies frequency-dependence. The in-phase component defines the dynamic elastic modulus,

$$E_{dyn} = |E_c| \cos\phi \qquad (3.1.22)$$

and the viscous modulus is defined by

$$\eta\omega = |E_c| \sin\phi \qquad (3.1.23)$$

where ϕ is the phase lag, generally between pressure (p) and diameter (D). In the case that pressure leads diameter, or that the diameter distention delays after the arrival of the pressure pulse, ϕ is positive. When the artery is assumed purely elastic, i.e. no viscosity damping is present, the arterial lumen diameter then changes instantaneously with the distending pressure pulse. In this case, φ is zero and the viscous term ηω disappears, as sin (0) = 0.

A similar form of complex elastic modulus was given by Cox (1975), accounting for arterial wall thickness:

$$E(\omega) = \frac{4a^2b}{b^2 - a^2} \frac{P(\omega)}{D(\omega)}$$ (3.1.24)

where *a* and *b* are inner and outer arterial diameters, respectively. P(ω) and D(ω) are frequency domain pressure and diameter, respectively.

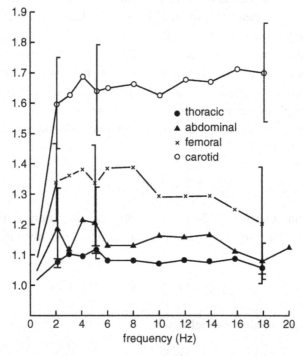

Fig. 3.1.3: Dynamic elastic modulus (E_{dyn}) plotted as a function of frequency for the thoracic aorta, abdominal aorta, femoral and carotid arteries. Notice the E_{dyn} is essentially unchanged above 2 Hz.

Experimental results show that the viscous modulus is small compared with the elastic modulus (Li *et al.*, 1981; Li, 1987; Nichols and O'Rourke, 1998). It is of the order of 10%. The dynamic modulus has also been found to be essentially constant above 2 Hz (Li, 2000). Similar frequency dependence is also seen in the "true phase velocity", discussed in more detail in Chapter 4.

A complex Young's modulus was considered by Westerhof and Noordergraaf (1970) to describe arterial wall viscoelasticity, also utilized frequency dependent parameters. They defined the complex elastic modulus as the ratio of complex stress to complex strain:

$$Ec(\omega) = \frac{\sigma(\omega)}{\varepsilon(\omega)} \qquad (3.1.25)$$

$$Ec(\omega) = \frac{F(\omega) / A}{\Delta l(\omega) / l(\omega)} \qquad (3.1.26)$$

It is clear that at $\omega = 0$, or when the elastic modulus is frequency-independent, eqn. (3.1.25) reduces to eqn. (3.1.14). As an example, $F(\omega)$ can be considered as the sinusoidally applied force, $l(\omega)$ is the length, and $\Delta l(\omega)$ is the change in length. In Laplace notation, they showed that if a unit change in length in the form of a step function is applied to the Voigt model (Fig. 3.1.4), its force development (stress relaxation) is unbounded. When a unit change in force is applied to the Maxwell model (Fig. 3.1.4), its change in length (creep phenomenon) is unbounded. Thus, both models do not exactly represent the physical properties of blood vessels. This indicates that a single time constant alone is not necessarily sufficient to describe either the stress-relaxation or the creep phenomenon. However, both Maxwell and Voigt models remain the most commonly used representation of biological viscoelastic properties. Although adding more spring-dashpot elements (e.g. to 5, 7 or 9-elements) allow better approximation of pressure-diameter or force-length responses, they have limitations in identifying physiological correspondences.

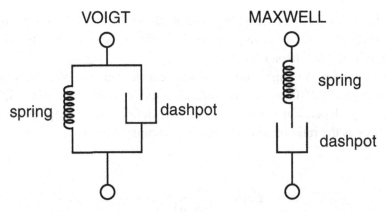

Fig. 3.1.4: Mechanical models of viscoelastic arteries. The spring-dashpot models are subjected to step changes in force, and step changes in length. In a Maxwell model (right), creep is unbounded; in a Voigt model (left), stress relaxation is unbounded.

3.2 Frequency Domain and Fourier Analysis

3.2.1 *Blood Pressure as a Periodic Function*

A periodic function with a period T, is defined by

$$f(t) = f(t + T) \qquad (3.2.1)$$

And it follows that:

$$f(t) = f(t + nT), n = 0, \pm 1, \pm 2, \dots \qquad (3.2.2)$$

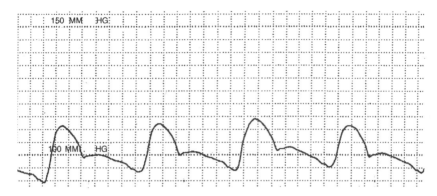

Fig. 3.2.1: Measured aortic blood pressure waveforms showing periodicity. Oscillations within systolic and diastolic pressure levels are slightly modulated by respiratory effects.

Figure 3.2.1 illustrates the periodic blood pressure waveforms oscillating within systolic and diastolic pressure levels with cardiac period T. There is in general a slight change in pressure waveform amplitudes due to the influence of respiration, i.e. inspiration and expiration. In this case, we have for the pulsatile pressure waveforms:

$$p(t) = p(t + nT), n = 0, \pm 1, \pm 2, ... \qquad (3.2.3)$$

It is clear that any periodic signal satisfying the Dirichlet conditions (convergence conditions) can be expressed by the Fourier series. To apply the Fourier series, periodicity and linearity need to be satisfied. Periodicity is often observed, because cardiac period is varies little from beat to beat during a short interval.

3.2.2 *Trigonometric Fourier Series*

A periodic function can be expressed in terms of its sine and cosine components:

$$f(t) = a_0 + a_1 \cos \omega_0 t + a_2 \cos 2\omega_0 t + ... + b_1 \sin \omega_0 t + b_2 \sin 2\omega_0 t + ...$$

$$(3.2.4)$$

which is

$$f(t) = a_0 + \sum_{n=1}^{N} \left[(a_n \cos(n\omega_0 t) + b_n \sin(n\omega_0 t) \right] \qquad (3.2.5)$$

where the Fourier coefficients are:

$$a_0 = \frac{1}{T} \int_0^T f(t) dt \qquad (3.2.6)$$

$$a_n = \frac{2}{T} \int_0^T f(t) \cos(n\omega_0 t) dt \qquad (3.2.7)$$

$$b_n = \frac{2}{T} \int_0^T f(t) \sin(n\omega_0 t) dt \qquad (3.2.8)$$

$$\omega_0 = 2\pi f = \frac{2\pi}{T} \qquad (3.2.9)$$

where ω_0 is the angular frequency, f_0 is the fundamental frequency and T is the period, n is the nth number of harmonics and N is the total number of harmonics in the Fourier series summation.

The trigonometric representations of the above series give the following:

$$f(t) = c_0 + \sum_{n=1}^{N} c_n \cos(n\omega_0 t - \theta_n) \qquad (3.2.10)$$

where the harmonic magnitude and phase are represented by

$$c_n = \sqrt{a_n^2 + b_n^2} \qquad (3.2.11)$$

and

$$\theta_n = \tan^{-1}\frac{b_n}{a_n} \tag{3.2.12}$$

In terms of pulsatile pressure waveforms, the Fourier series can be written as:

$$p(t) = \overline{p} + \sum_{n=1}^{N} p_n \cos(n\omega t - \phi_n) \tag{3.2.13}$$

Thus, Fourier series representation of a periodic pressure waveform is the summation of a mean pressure component (first term) and its sinusoidal or co-sinusoidal harmonic components.

A similar Fourier series representation can be written for the flow waveform:

$$Q(t) = \overline{Q} + \sum_{n=1}^{N} Q_n \cos(n\omega t - \varphi_n) \tag{3.2.14}$$

Figure 3.2.2 gives an example of the summation of Fourier components that provides the resynthesis of the aortic pressure waveform. For the aortic pressure waveform, 10 harmonics are sufficient to accurately reconstruct the waveform.

3.2.3 Complex Form of Fourier Series

By expressing sine and cosine in terms of exponentials, we have

$$\cos(n\omega_0 t) = \frac{1}{2}(e^{jn\omega_0 t} + e^{-jn\omega_0 t}) \tag{3.2.15}$$

$$\sin(n\omega_0 t) = \frac{1}{2j}(e^{jn\omega_0 t} - e^{-jn\omega_0 t}) \tag{3.2.16}$$

and substituting into

$$f(t) = a_0 + \sum_{n=1}^{N}\left[(a_n \cos(n\omega_0 t) + b_n \sin(n\omega_0 t)\right] \tag{3.2.17}$$

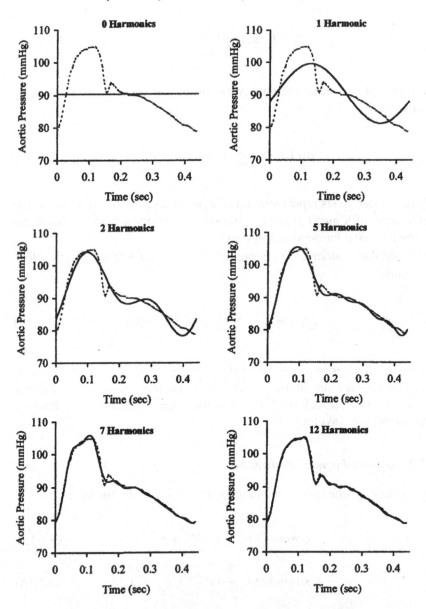

Fig. 3.2.2: Re-synthesis of aortic pressure waveform by summation of different number of harmonic components, up to the 12th. Ten harmonics are generally considered adequate to reconstruct accurately the aortic pressure waveform.

We have

$$f(t) = \frac{1}{2}a_0 + \sum_{n=1}^{N}\left[\frac{1}{2}(a_n - jb_n)e^{jn\omega_0 t} + \frac{1}{2}(a_n + jb_n)e^{-jn\omega_0 t}\right] \quad (3.2.18)$$

or simply:

$$f(t) = c_0 + \sum_{n=1}^{N}(c_n e^{jn\omega_0 t} + c_{-n}e^{-jn\omega_0 t}) \quad (3.2.19)$$

where

$$c_0 = \frac{1}{2}a_0 = \frac{1}{T}\int_0^T f(t)dt \quad (3.2.20)$$

$$c_n = \frac{1}{2}(a_n - jb_n) = \frac{1}{T}\int_0^T f(t)e^{-jn\omega_0 t}dt \quad (3.2.21)$$

$$c_{-n} = \frac{1}{2}(a_n + jb_n) = \frac{1}{T}\int_0^T f(t)e^{jn\omega_0 t}dt \quad (3.2.22)$$

For real f(t), then c_{-n} is c_n's complex conjugate, and if phase is considered, then:

$$c_n = |c_n|e^{j(n\omega_0 t - \theta_n)} \quad (3.2.23)$$

where

$$|c_n| = \frac{1}{2}\sqrt{a_n^2 + b_n^2} \quad (3.2.24)$$

and

$$\theta_n = \tan^{-1}(\frac{-b_n}{a_n}) \quad (3.2.25)$$

In terms of pulsatile blood pressure waveforms p(t), we have for mean pressure:

$$\bar{p} = \frac{1}{T}\int_0^T p(t)dt \qquad (3.2.26)$$

and for the nth harmonic of the pressure waveform:

$$P_n(\omega) = |P_n(\omega)|e^{j(n\omega_0 t - \phi_n)} \qquad (3.2.27)$$

For the corresponding flow waveform harmonic component, we have

$$Q_n(\omega) = |Q_n(\omega)|e^{j(n\omega_0 t - \varphi_n)} \qquad (3.2.28)$$

Vascular impedance, expressed as the harmonic ratios of pressure to flow, is:

$$Z_n(\omega) = |Z_n(\omega)|e^{j\theta_n} \qquad (3.2.29)$$

From which, it is clear that the magnitude and phase for the corresponding harmonics are

$$|Z_n| = \frac{|P_n|}{|Q_n|} \quad \text{and} \quad \theta_n = \phi_n - \varphi_n \qquad (3.2.30)$$

3.2.4 *Other Aspects of Frequency Domain Analysis*

3.2.4.1 Dirichlet Conditions

We have assumed that in the forgoing discussions that a periodic function, and the pressure and flow waveforms can be represented by the Fourier series. In general, there is a convergence requirement that is known as the Dirichlet Conditions, under which a Fourier series representation of a function f(t) is possible. The Dirichlet conditions are as follows:

(1) the function f(t) has a finite number of discontinuities in one period,

(2) the function f(t) has a finite number of maxima and minima in one period,

(3) the function f(t) is absolutely integrable over a period.

The function is said to be piecewise continuous in the finite interval T if conditions (1) and (2) are satisfied.

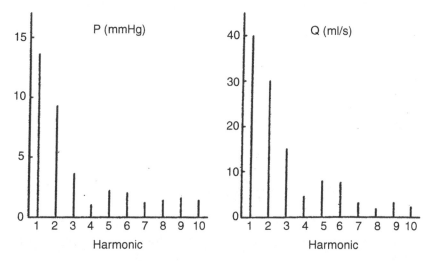

Fig. 3.2.3: Harmonic magnitudes of an aortic pressure pulse (mmHg) and an aortic flow pulse (ml/s).

3.2.4.2 Line Spectrum and Nyquist Criterion

The harmonic magnitudes of a typical aortic pressure pulse and aortic flow pulse are shown in Fig. 3.2.3. The magnitudes are small and negligible beyond the tenth harmonic component. The Nyquist criterion requires sampling frequency of at least twice the highest frequency content in order to reconstruct the original waveform accurately. In the present example, for a heart rate of 90 beats/min or 1.5 Hz, the tenth harmonic would be 15 Hz. The minimal sampling frequency required is therefore 30 Hz. In most cases, sampling frequency applied is much higher than this and typically at 100Hz. In other words, the pressure waveform is digitized at 10 msec intervals.

3.2.4.3 Correlation, Coherence and Power Spectrum

Autocorrelation for a periodic function f(t) can be defined by

$$\frac{1}{T}\int_0^T f_1(t)f_1(t+\tau)dt = \sum_0^\infty \left|F(n\omega)_1\right|^2 e^{jn\omega\tau} \qquad (3.2.31)$$

where τ represents the time delay. Its power spectrum is given as

$$\Phi_{11}(n\omega) = \left|F_1(n\omega)\right|^2 \qquad (3.2.32)$$

$$\phi_{11}(\tau) = \sum_0^\infty \Phi_{11}(n\omega)e^{jn\omega\tau} \qquad (3.2.33)$$

and inversely,

$$\Phi_{11}(n\omega) = \frac{1}{T}\int_0^T \phi_{11}(\tau)e^{-jn\omega\tau} \qquad (3.2.34)$$

Similarly, the cross-correlation for two functions $f_1(t)$ and $f_2(t)$ can be defined as:

$$\phi_{12}(\tau) = \frac{1}{T}\int_0^T f_1(t)f_2(t+\tau)dt = \sum_0^\infty \left|F_{12}(n\omega)_1\right|^2 e^{jn\omega\tau} \qquad (3.2.35)$$

$$\phi_{12}(\tau) = \sum_0^\infty \Phi_{12}(n\omega)e^{jn\omega\tau} \qquad (3.2.36)$$

and

$$\Phi_{12}(n\omega) = \frac{1}{T}\int_0^T \phi_{12}(\tau)e^{-jn\omega\tau} \qquad (3.2.37)$$

which has a co-spectral of C_{12} and quadrature term, Q_{12}.

As an example, given that pressure and flow can be represented by $f_1(t)$ and $f_2(t)$, we have for impedance:

$$Z = |Z|e^{-j\theta}$$

(3.2.38)

which can be written as

$$|Z| = \sqrt{\frac{\Phi_{11}}{\Phi_{12}}}$$

(3.2.39)

with a phase

$$\theta = \tan^{-1}\frac{Q_{12}}{C_{12}}$$

(3.2.40)

The coherence observed is given by

$$C_{oe} = \frac{(C_{12}^{2} + Q_{12}^{2})}{\sqrt{\Phi_{11} \cdot \Phi_{12}}}$$

(3.2.41)

3.3 Fluid Mechanics and Rheology

3.3.1 *Steady Flow, the Poiseuille Equation and Flow Velocity Profile*

The flow of viscous blood in a relatively cylindrical elastic arterial vessel has borrowed much of the quantitative treatment from fluid mechanics. Navier-Stokes equations are the fundamental equations describing fluid motion. Poiseuille equation is a special case of the general solution of the Navier-Stokes equations.

Steady pressure-flow relations are commonly described by the Poiseuille's equation:

$$Q = \frac{\pi r^{4}\Delta p}{8\eta l}$$

(3.3.1)

where Q is the mean or steady flow in ml/s, r is the inner radius of the vessel, l is the length through which blood flows and η is the viscosity of the fluid, in this case, blood (0.03 poise or 3 centi-poise) and Δp is the pressure drop across the vessel. Thus, the amount of flow is critically dependent on the size of the lumen radius and is proportional to its fourth power. This equation has also been used to determine fluid viscosity, by measuring flow and pressure drop over a known geometry of the tube. The Poiseuille resistance, Rs, to steady flow is seen as the ratio of Δp/Q or simply equals to $8\eta l/\pi r^4$.

The force opposing the flow of a viscous fluid with surface area A, is proportional to the viscosity and the velocity gradient (v/d) across the fluid layers with separation d. This defines the fluid viscosity as,

$$\eta = \frac{F/A}{v/d} \tag{3.3.2}$$

It is clear that the numerator is the applied pressure and the denominator, velocity gradient. Thus, the more viscous the fluid, the greater amount of pressure is needed to apply to the fluid to generate the same amount of velocity gradient. Blood thinner or the popularly used low dosage (81mg) aspirin is to temporarily reduce blood viscosity, thus allowing more relief blood flow. This has been found to have long-term benefits as well for the cardiac patients.

For a constant vessel geometry and fluid viscosity, it can be seen that the pressure gradient governs the flow. From Fig. 3.3.1, it is clear that the pressure gradient is

$$\frac{dp}{dz} \approx \frac{\Delta p}{\Delta z} \approx \frac{(p_1 - p_2)}{l} \tag{3.3.3}$$

For pulsatile flow, this pressure gradient changes with time. In fact, before the advent of electromagnetic and ultrasonic flow transducers, derivation of flow from pressure gradient was common. This latter was applied to obtain pulsatile flow information, rather the steady or mean flow.

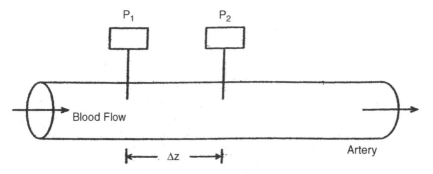

Fig. 3.3.1: A cylindrical tube containing steady flow of a fluid with viscosity η. Two pressures, p_1 and p_2 measured at finite distance Δz apart allow pressure gradient $\Delta p/\Delta z$ to be calculated.

The velocity profile for a steady, laminar flow is based on the general derivation of Poiseuille's equation. Consider a cylindrical vessel with internal radius r_i and length l, the viscous force exerted on the cylindrical unit of fluid is (with p=F/A and circular cross-sectional area, $A=\pi r^2$):

$$F_p = (p_1 - p_2)\pi r^2 \qquad (3.3.4)$$

The viscous force retarding the motion of the cylindrical volume of flow, is, from (3.3.2), the product of cross-sectional area and viscosity, multiplied by the velocity gradient,

$$F_\eta = 2\pi r l \eta \frac{dv}{dr} \qquad (3.3.5)$$

Under equilibrium, these forces balance each other, i.e. equal and opposite,

$$(p_1 - p_2)\pi r^2 = -2\pi r l \eta \frac{dv}{dr} \qquad (3.3.6)$$

The velocity gradient for the particular laminar layer of fluid is therefore,

$$\frac{dv}{dr} = -\frac{(p_1 - p_2)}{2\eta l} \tag{3.3.7}$$

Substituting for the pressure gradient from equation (3.3.3), we have the relation between the velocity gradient and pressure gradient,

$$\frac{dv}{dr} = -\frac{1}{2\eta}\frac{dp}{dz} \tag{3.3.8}$$

Notice that the velocity gradient is in the radial direction, i.e. across the vessel, whereas the pressure gradient is in the longitudinal direction, i.e. along the vessel axis. Velocity at radius r across the vessel can be readily obtained by integration of (3.3.7)

$$v = -\frac{(p_1 - p_2)r^2}{4\eta l} + k \tag{3.3.9}$$

where k is the constant of integration, obtainable by applying the boundary condition that the velocity of fluid at the vessel wall ($r=r_i$) is zero, i.e. $v(r=r_i) = 0$. We have,

$$v = \frac{1}{4\eta}\frac{(p_1 - p_2)}{l}(r_i^2 - r^2) \tag{3.3.10}$$

Thus, velocity is maximum, or v_{max}, when r=0, or along the axis,

$$v_{max} = \frac{(p_1 - p_2)r_i^2}{4\eta l} \tag{3.3.11}$$

This is sometimes referred to as the centerline velocity or axial velocity. The velocity is zero at the vessel wall, when $r=r_i$.

Equation (3.3.10) is that of a parabola, hence the velocity profile across the vessel wall is known as a parabolic velocity profile. This is shown in Fig. 3.3.2.

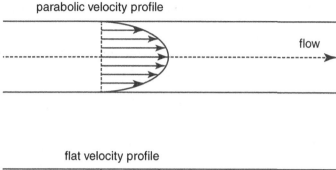

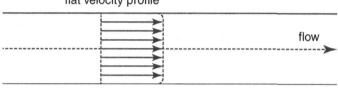

Fig. 3.3.2: Illustration of two different velocity profiles. Top: the velocity is maximal at the centerline and decreases progressively towards the vessel wall in a parabolic fashion. Bottom: a flat velocity profile where velocity is uniformly high across the lumen.

The amount of flow, or volume flow, is obtained as,

$$Q = \int_0^{r_i} 2\pi r v \, dr \qquad (3.3.12)$$

which results in the well-known Poiseuille equation

$$Q = \frac{\pi r_i^4 (p_1 - p_2)}{8\eta l} \qquad (3.3.13)$$

The average velocity across the velocity profile is simply the amount of flow divide by the cross-sectional area of the vessel lumen, πr_i^2,

$$v_{av} = \frac{r^2}{8\eta l}(p_1 - p_2) \qquad (3.3.14)$$

3.3.2 *Bernoulli's Equation and Narrowing Vessel Lumen or Stenosis*

For a vessel with a narrowed segment or stenosis, as shown in Fig. 3.3.3, the total volume flow through all segments must be the same, by the conservation of mass. The flow is given by the product of the cross-sectional area and the flow velocity:

$$Q = A_1 v_1 = A_2 v_2 = A_3 v_3 \qquad (3.3.15)$$

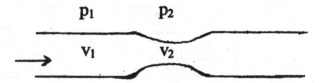

Fig. 3.3.3: A cylindrical vessel with a narrowed segment or stenosis. Greater the pressure drop (p_1-p_2), results in faster flow velocity through the stenosis, v_2, compared with pre-stenotic velocity v_1. Post-stenotic dilation is often observed.

The familiar kinetic energy equation is given as

$$K.E. = \frac{1}{2} m v^2 \qquad (3.3.16)$$

and the corresponding potential energy is

$$P.E. = pQ \qquad (3.3.17)$$

The total energy is their sum:

$$W = P.E. + K.E. \qquad (3.3.18)$$

This gives rise to

$$W_1 = (h\rho g)(A_1 v_1) + \frac{1}{2}(\rho A_1 v_1) v_1^2 \qquad (3.3.19)$$

associated with the pre-stenotic section, with $p=h\rho g$ due to gravity or static pressure difference.

We have also, for the stenotic section:

$$W_2 = (h\rho g)(A_2 v_2) + \frac{1}{2}(\rho A_2 v_2)v_2^{\,2} \qquad (3.3.20)$$

From the conservation of energy, equating these 2 equations, we have

$$(p_1 - p_2) + \frac{1}{2}\rho(v_1^{\,2} - v_2^{\,2}) + \rho g(h_1 - h_2) = k \qquad (3.3.21)$$

For the case when gravity is ignored or when $h_1=h_2$, we have the familiar Bernoulli equation

$$p_1 = p_2 + \frac{1}{2}\rho(v_1^{\,2} - v_2^{\,2}) \qquad (3.3.22)$$

The commonly known phrase that the faster the flow velocity, the lower the pressure, i.e. $v_2 > v_1$, then $p_2 < p_1$. This is clearly seen from the illustration in the figure. The well-known Bernoulli equation described above is for a steady, inviscid (non-viscous) and incompressible fluid flow.

3.3.3 Orifice Flow and Torricelli's Equation

The problem of flow through an orifice small in dimension compared with the reservoir was considered by Torricelli in the 17th century. The pressure and velocity at the surface of the reservoir are p_1 and v_1 and those at the orifice are p_2 and v_2, respectively. We have for the velocities,

$$v_2^{\,2} - v_1^{\,2} = \frac{2}{\rho}(p_1 - p_2) + 2g(h_1 - h_2) \qquad (3.3.23)$$

From continuity equation that flow entering equals flow leaving, we have

$$v_1 A_1 = v_2 A_2 \qquad (3.3.24)$$

In general, $A_1 >> A_2$ and $v_1 << v_2$ and assume $p_1 = p_2$, we have

$$v_2^2 = 2g(h_1 - h_2) \qquad (3.3.25)$$

This results in the Torricelli's equation describing the velocity speed of flow leaving the orifice. Substituting $v = v_2$, we obtain

$$v = \sqrt{2g(h_1 - h_2)} \qquad (3.3.26)$$

The amount of flow leaving the orifice with circular cross section of radius r is therefore,

$$Q = \pi r^2 v = \pi r^2 \sqrt{2g(h_1 - h_2)} \qquad (3.3.27)$$

3.3.4 *Valvular Cross-section and the Gorlin Equation*

A popular equation that has been used in the clinical applications is the Gorlin equation describing the orifice cross-section area. The equation is used in calculating valvular cross-sectional area, particularly during valvular stenostic conditions. The orifice cross-sectional area is given by:

$$A = \frac{Q}{\sqrt{2g(p_1 - p_2)}} \frac{1}{\pi K_c} \qquad (3.3.28)$$

where K_c is the contraction coefficient or the ratio of the cross-sectional area of orifice flow jet to the actual opening of the orifice

$$K_c = A_o / A \qquad (3.3.29)$$

3.3.5 *Flow and Flow Acceleration*

The Cartesian coordinates in three dimensions, in the x-axis, y-axis and z-axis together with time is usually represented as:

$$f = f(x, y, z, t) \qquad (3.3.30)$$

The cylindrical polar coordinates representation, one has

$$f = f(z, r, \theta, t) \qquad (3.3.31)$$

Thus for velocities, u, v, w, we have

$$u = u(z, r, \theta, t)$$
$$v = v(z, r, \theta, t) \qquad (3.3.32)$$
$$w = w(z, r, \theta, t)$$

along the direction of flow z in a cylindrical blood vessel, along its radius (r) or radial component, and the rotational component associated with an angular component (θ). This representation identifies position within the blood vessel at any given time t. This coordinates system was originated by Euler, and is sometimes referred to as the Eulerian velocities.

Thus, it is clear that when the positions are time-dependent, i.e. the fluid element moves from one position to another with changing time, we have, for the velocities:

$$u = \frac{dz}{dt}$$
$$v = \frac{dr}{dt} \qquad (3.3.33)$$
$$w = r\frac{d\theta}{dt}$$

Velocity is clearly seen here defined as the rate of change of distance traveled or position. In the case of irrotational flow, or that the rotational flow component is negligible, one remains with u and v. In the case of one-dimensional flow, i.e. along the longitudinal z-axis of the vessel then only u exists.

The rate of change of flow velocity is the acceleration. Faster rate of change in velocity gives rise to a greater acceleration in flow. Such acceleration can be either positive, i.e. when the velocity is increasing or negative, i.e. when the velocity is reducing. This can be appreciated from the aortic flow velocity recording and its derivative. Figure 3.3.4 shows the aortic flow and the flow acceleration, together with simultaneously recorded aortic pressure and its first derivative. Peak flow acceleration, and maximum pressure derivative have both been used as an index of cardiac contractility. Thus, faster the aortic flow acceleration during the ejection phase, the stronger the cardiac contraction.

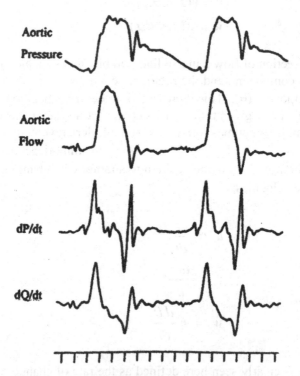

Fig. 3.3.4: Aortic flow and its first derivative, the flow acceleration (dQ/dt). Aortic pressure and rate of its pressure change (dP/dt) is also shown.

Thus acceleration is the rate of change of velocity. We have for the accelerations associated with the longitudinal, radial and rotational velocities (Noordergraaf, 1969):

$$a_z = \frac{\partial u}{\partial t} + u \frac{\partial u}{\partial z} + v \frac{\partial u}{\partial r} + \frac{w}{r} \frac{\partial u}{\partial \theta}$$

$$a_r = \frac{\partial v}{\partial t} + u \frac{\partial v}{\partial z} + v \frac{\partial v}{\partial r} + \frac{w}{r} \frac{\partial v}{\partial \theta} - \frac{w}{r^2} \qquad (3.3.34)$$

$$a_\theta = \frac{\partial w}{\partial t} + u \frac{\partial w}{\partial z} + v \frac{\partial w}{\partial r} + \frac{w}{r} \frac{\partial w}{\partial \theta} + \frac{vw}{r}$$

These partial derivatives of velocities other than the first terms are sometimes known as convective accelerations. Notice that acceleration at a particular instant in time when z, r, and θ, are kept constant (i.e. velocities do not change with z, r and θ), one obtains the familiar equations for acceleration:

$$a_z = \frac{\partial u}{\partial t}$$

$$a_r = \frac{\partial v}{\partial t} \qquad (3.3.35)$$

$$a_\theta = \frac{\partial w}{\partial t}$$

3.3.6 *Newtonian Fluid, No-Slip, Boundary Conditions and Entry Length*

3.3.6.1 Newtonian Fluid

The coefficient of viscosity of blood as we have shown earlier, is defined as the ratio of applied pressure to the velocity gradient. In other words, it is the shear stress that represents the resisting force of the fluid deformation along the direction of flow:

$$\tau_s = \eta \frac{dv}{dz} \qquad (3.3.36)$$

Fluid that behaves in this manner is known as the Newtonian fluid, attributed to its originator, Newton. This assumes that the rate of deformation, or the velocity gradient is small. And for a cylindrical vessel with velocity v, and diameter d, this becomes:

$$\eta = \frac{F/A}{v/d} \qquad (3.3.37)$$

Blood has plasma, blood cells and other formed elements. In most common analysis of blood flow in vessels, the assumption of blood as a Newtonian fluid seems to work well. Except in the case of very small vessels, such as the small arterioles capillaries where red blood cell size actually approaches that of the vessel lumen diameter, one needs to be concerned, not only of fluid shear, but also of shear stress on the flowing red blood cell and of the differential velocity gradients generated by the formed elements.

3.3.6.2 No-Slip Boundary Conditions

The "no-slip" condition refers to the assumption that concerns the fluid-solid interface or blood-vessel wall interface. No-slip boundary condition refers to the condition when the flow velocity at the tube wall is the same as the wall velocity, such that there is no "jump' or a step change in velocity to cause discontinuity. The general assumption is that the fluid in contact with the wall does not move at all. This assumption is generally true for the large vessels. In small vessels, plasma dominates as fluid and this no-slip condition generally applies to the plasma in contact with the wall, rather than red blood cells or the formed elements in blood.

3.3.6.3 Laminar and Turbulent Flow

Reynolds apparently was the first to use dye of visible color to investigate the manner in which fluid flows in a tube and provided a quantitative relation between the viscosity of the fluid and the mass of the fluid. Reynolds number as it is called, and as we derived earlier is given by

$$R_e = \frac{\rho v d}{\eta}$$

(3.3.38)

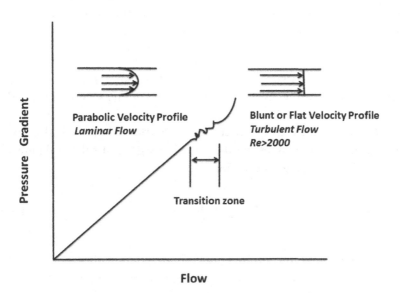

Fig. 3.3.5: Illustration of laminar to turbulent flow transition as a function of Reynolds number. Velocity transition from a parabolic profile to a blunt profile is also seen (see also Fig. 3.3.2).

The most important observation and quantification made by Reynolds is in the differentiation of turbulent flow from laminar flow. This means that the turbulence depends not only on the average velocity v of the fluid, but also depending on the fluid property and the lumen diameter d.

The laminar to turbulent flow transition is shown in Fig. 3.3.5. Reynolds number of 2000 is assumed when turbulence begins. The Mach number is invariant among mammalian blood vessels, but the

Reynolds number is dependent on body size (Li, 2000). Turbulence that normally occurs with high Reynolds number is somewhat constrained in a larger mammal's aorta by the larger compliance (Li, 1988).

3.3.6.4 Entry Length

Entry length is defined as the distance from the entrance or inlet of a vessel at which point the flow is fully developed. In the case of Poiseuille flow, this means that the centerline velocity reaches its maximum with the velocity profile becomes fully parabolic. But Poiseuille flow assumes a tube that is long enough for such flow to occur. However, under pulsatile flow conditions, flow does not fully develop and hence the accuracy in the determination of entry length becomes an issue. This is normally circumvented by assuming that the flow is almost fully developed in analyzing flow in blood vessels. A common criterion that is used assumes that the centerline velocity is within 1 or 2% of the centerline velocity according to Poiseuille's flow, i.e. 98% or 99%.

The determined entry length is of course determined also by the manner in which flow enters the vessel. A general rule of thumb used follows the following formulation:

$$\frac{l_e}{d} = 0.04 R_e \qquad\qquad (3.3.39)$$

This assumes that the entry length l_e in a vessel of diameter d as a flow with uniform velocity v. R_e is Reynolds number, as defined above.

Because of the finite geometry of the vascular segments, i.e. finite length and diameter, there are situation where the entry length requirement for an almost fully developed flow is not met. Thus, flow is frequently accepted as partially developed. A lower Reynolds number, such as those occurring at smaller vessels, with much smaller lumen diameters, the requirement of the entry length becomes much less stringent.

Chapter 4

Hemodynamics of Arteries

4.1 Blood Pressure and Flow Relations

4.1.1 *Pulsatile Pressure and Flow Waveforms in Arteries*

Pressure and flow waveforms in different anatomic locations in the vascular system owe to their structural and geometric nonuniformities, as well as central and peripheral interactions. Simultaneous recordings of pressure and flow waveforms in different parts of the vascular tree have shown some distinct features as the pulse travels away from the heart. First, the pressure pulse increases and the flow pulse decreases in amplitude progressively. The mean blood pressure declines slowly in arteries, but dramatically so in the arteriolar beds, as seen in Chapter 2. Secondly, the rate of rise of the pressure (dp/dt) in early systole increases and the wavefront becomes steeper, while that of the flow wave behaves in just the opposite manner. Thirdly, the incisura, or dicrotic notch, due to aortic valve closure, is more rounded as the pressure wave propagates towards the periphery and the diastolic pressure wave becomes more accentuated. These features are seen from Fig. 4.1.1. These observed changes are related to the functional aspects of the arterial system. Consequently, considerable diagnostic information can be derived from the accurate measurements and analysis of pressure and flow pulse contours. This makes pulse waveform analysis (PWA) an important tool in research and in clinical diagnostic settings.

Multi-sensor catheter has been used for simultaneous recordings of pressure and flow waveforms at several sites along the pulse propagation path. This allows extraction of pulse transmission information and in the interpretation of hemodynamic alterations in diseased conditions.

Simultaneous recording of pressure and flow velocity waveforms in man can be achieved in the clinical setting with catheter tip pressure and velocity sensors. In general, pressure as well as flow waveforms are similar at corresponding anatomic sites among many mammalian species (Li and Noordergaaf, 1991; Li, 1996).

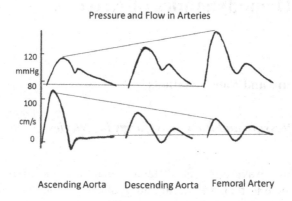

Fig. 4.1.1: Pressure and flow waveforms in the ascending aorta, descending aorta and the femoral artery. Away from the heart, the progressive increases in pulse pressure and decreases in pulsatile flow magnitudes are seen.

Blood pressure waveforms are periodical, as illustrated in Fig. 4.1.2 which displays pressure waveforms recorded in the ascending aorta, descending thoracic aorta, the abdominal aorta and the iliac artery, when the catheter-tip pressure transducer is slowly withdrawn away from the heart. The progressive increases in pulse pressure amplitudes with increasing systolic pressure and decreasing diastolic pressure can be observed. The electrocardiogram (ECG) is normally recorded as timing reference and for the calculation of cardiac period (T). The bottom tracing is the ascending aortic flow measured with an electromagnetic flow probe. The waveforms are reproducible following each heartbeat. This is normally true under steady state conditions.

Respiratory influence on the pressure waveforms is easily observed when consecutive beats are recorded over a respiratory cycle. The normal ratio of heart frequency to respiratory frequency is about 4 to 1.

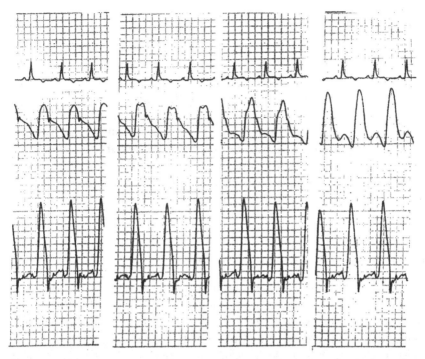

Fig. 4.1.2: Simultaneously recorded electrocardiogram (top panel), blood pressure (middle panel) and ascending aortic flow (bottom panel) waveforms. Pressure waveforms in the ascending aorta (first left), descending thoracic aorta (second left), the abdominal aorta (second right) and the iliac artery (first right) are shown.

The changes induced by respiration are usually small, except in some pathological conditions, such as in pulsus paradoxus where blood pressure changes are excessive during both inspiration and expiration.

The more distal the pressure pulse away from the heart, the larger is its amplitude. This is attributed to the larger amplitudes of peripheral wave reflections. Such reflections have been suggested as a closed-end type, with the principal sites of reflections in the arterioles. Structural and geometric changes along a vessel also give rise to reflections, but are of smaller magnitudes. Reflections, in general, have opposite effects on pressure and flow.

Geometric nonuniformities constitute the second factor that influences the pulse waveforms. These may be tapering or vascular branching. The many aspects of vascular branching are the subject of the following chapter.

The third influential factor is elastic nonuniformity. The vascular wall becomes progressively stiffer toward the periphery owing to increased elastic moduli, and accounts for the dispersion of wave velocity.

Finally, the wall and fluid viscosities attenuate the pulse wave. The extent of attenuation, or the degree of damping, is greater at higher frequencies. For instance, the pulse at the femoral artery no longer exhibits the characteristic high frequency features of the aortic pulse. Instead, a smooth waveform is seen. The pulse reaching the arterioles is normally so damped that its waveform appears sinusoidal.

In summary, pressure and flow pulses are modified as they travel away from the heart due to (1) wave reflections, (2) geometric nonuniformity, (3) elastic nonuniformity, and (4) damping.

4.1.2 *Pressure-flow Relations in the Aorta*

At the onset of systole, left ventricular pressure (LVP or Pv) develops rapidly during the cardiac isometric contraction period. When LVP exceeds the aortic pressure (AoP or Pa), ventricular ejection begins. The ventricular outflow is large and rapid at the onset of ejection, becomes more gradual and then declines towards end-systole. At aortic valve closure, there is backflow, followed by small oscillations. In diastole, the aortic flow reaches zero. The diastolic aortic pressure decays precipitously towards end-diastole. In the Windkessel approximation, this decay follows a mono-exponential pattern. In actuality, there are oscillations superimposed on the diastolic pressure and the decay is not necessarily mono-exponential.

The right ventricle and the pulmonary arterial system are known as the "low pressure" system and the left ventricle and the systemic arterial system are known as the "high pressure" system. This implies that pulmonary aorta has a much lower pressure amplitude that that of the aorta. The stroke volumes are the same, therefore, the flow magnitudes are similar, although their waveforms can be quite different. Figure 4.1.3 illustrates the differences. The pulmonary aorta is much more compliant than the aorta and the pressure waveform tends to be more closer in morphology to the flow waveform (Van den Bos *et al.*, 1982). This has been attributed to the comparatively smaller amount of wave reflections in the pulmonary system. This is due to the spatial distribution of compliances that are greater in the pulmonary arteries than the stiffer systemic arteries.

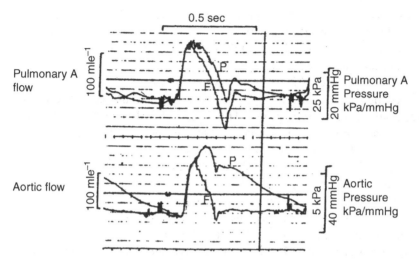

Fig. 4.1.3: Simultaneously recorded pressure and flow waveforms in the pulmonary aorta (top tracings) and in the ascending aorta (bottom tracings). Notice the pressure and flow waveforms are more similar in the more compliant pulmonary arterial system. Peak flow waveform corresponds to inflection point on the early systolic pressure waveform.

The inflection point corresponding to blood pressure at which peak flow occurs is higher in the pulmonary aorta, indicating a smaller augmented pressure (peak systolic pressure-inflection pressure or Ps-Pi), than that in the systemic aorta. Some have interpreted this as a higher wave reflection in the early systole in the systemic aorta. Major reflections from the peripheral sites do not reach the proximal aortas in the early ejection phase in any appreciable fashion. Thus, the time courses of pressure and flow waveforms are quite similar during this interval. The ventricles exert significance influence on the features of the aortic pressure and flow waveforms. The reverse is also true. This aspect of heart-arterial system interaction is presented in Chapter 9.

4.2 Vascular Impedance to Blood Flow

4.2.1 *The Impedance Concept and Formulation*

Under steady flow conditions, fluid resistance can be readily calculated from the Poiseuille formula. When pressure and flow are oscillatory and periodic under pulsatile conditions, frequency dependent impedance representation is necessary.

The impedance of the total systemic vascular tree, or the input impedance to the arterial system, is defined as the complex ratio by harmonic of pressure to flow. This is so defined when the pressure and flow waveforms are measured at the entrance to the arterial system, namely, at the root or the aorta or ascending aorta. This is the vascular load that the heart "sees" during ejection, as input to the arterial system (hence termed the "input impedance" of the arterial system). Impedance can also be measured at different parts of the circulation. For instance, when pressure and flow are measured at the femoral artery, then the vascular impedance so obtained represents that of the impedance of the femoral arterial vascular bed. Similarly, there can be renal arterial impedance and cerebral vascular impedance. Each governs the blood flow going into their vascular beds.

Vascular impedance has both a magnitude and a phase associated with each individual harmonic component. Since pressure and flow are generally not in phase, the impedance possesses a phase angle within 90°. This is attributed to the time delayed arrival between the pressure pulse and the flow pulse at an arterial site. When the particular pressure harmonic leads the flow harmonic, then the phase angle between them is positive. Conversely, when the pressure harmonic lags behind the corresponding flow harmonic, then the phase is negative. Phase difference in the frequency domain, therefore, refers to time delay in the time domain.

The harmonic contents of pressure and flow waveforms can be obtained through Fourier analysis, as discussed in Chapter 3. Pulsatile blood pressure waveform can be considered an oscillatory part with sinusoidal components oscillating at different harmonic frequencies, $n\omega$, and phase, ϕ_n, superimposed on a DC component or mean blood pressure:

$$p(t) = \overline{p} + \sum_{n=1}^{N} p_n \sin(n\omega t + \phi_n) \qquad (4.2.1)$$

$$\omega = 2\pi f \tag{4.2.2}$$

where f (Hz) is the number of heart beats per second. Similar equations can be written for the flow waveform.

The relations for the pressure and flow pulse waveforms expressed as magnitude and phase are, for the nth harmonic:

$$P_n = \left|P_n\right| e^{j(\omega t + \phi_n)} \tag{4.2.3}$$

$$Q = \left|Q_n\right| e^{j(\omega t + \varphi_n)} \tag{4.2.4}$$

The ratio of pressure to flow is, therefore,

$$\frac{P}{Q} = \frac{\left|P_n\right| e^{j(\omega t + \phi_n)}}{\left|Q_n\right| e^{j(\omega t + \varphi_n)}} \tag{4.2.5}$$

The vascular impedance obtained for the nth harmonic is therefore

$$Z_n = \left|Z_n\right| e^{j\theta_n} \tag{4.2.6}$$

where the magnitude of impedance is simply the ratio of the pressure amplitude to the flow amplitude for the nth harmonic:

$$\left|Z_n\right| = \frac{\left|P_n\right|}{\left|Q_n\right|} \tag{4.2.7}$$

and the phase lag

$$\theta_n = \phi_n - \varphi_n \tag{4.2.8}$$

Pressure and flow waveforms do not necessarily contain the exact number of significant harmonics, as their waveforms and hence frequency contents differ. When the flow harmonic becomes very small, the ratio of pressure to flow or the impedance modulus for that harmonic component obtained can be erroneous.

4.2.2 Input Impedance and Characteristic Impedance

Input impedance of the systemic arterial tree has been obtained in the systemic and pulmonary, as well as the coronary arterial circulations. Vascular impedances have been measured in man, dog and other mammalian species. Figure 4.2.1 gives an example of the modulus of the vascular impedance measured at the ascending aorta or the input impedance to the systemic arterial tree in normal adults.

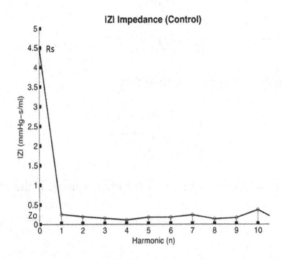

Fig. 4.2.1: Modulus of the impedance measured at the ascending aorta or input impedance of the systemic arterial tree. Rs refers to the total peripheral resistance. Z_0 indicates characteristic impedance of the proximal aorta.

Input impedance shows a large decrease in magnitude at very low frequencies (<2 Hz), then oscillates, exhibiting maxima and minima, and eventually reaches a somewhat constant level-low compared to its zero frequency (DC) value, at higher frequencies (>5 Hz). The input impedance (Z) approaches the characteristic impedance (Z_0) of the proximal aorta at these high frequencies. The phase of the impedance is initially negative, indicating flow leads pressure, becoming progressively more positive and crossing zero at about 3-5 Hz, and remains positive but close to zero thereafter. The characteristic maxima and minima associated with the input impedance spectrum are closely related to repeated and multi-site reflections in the arterial system (Berger *et al.*, 1993; Lei *et al.*, 1996).

The initial large decrease in impedance modulus accompanying a negative phase indicates that the load facing the left ventricle at low frequencies is capacitive in nature; recall that impedance due to a capacitive component is $Z(C)=1/j\omega C$ (Li, 2000). While at high frequencies it is inductive $(Z(L)=j\omega L)$. Thus, compliance (capacitive) and inertia (inductive) components of the arterial system can be estimated at these respective frequencies. Thus, the three-element Windkessel model can easily be modified to a four-element model by adding the inertia component. The viscous losses in the proximal aorta are small, but are more appreciable elsewhere in the arterial system (Li, 2000). Hence, approximating characteristic impedance by the high frequency values of the input impedance as a resistance is more accurate in the proximal aorta than in other smaller arteries.

$$Z_o \approx \overline{Z}(\omega)_{HF} \qquad (4.2.9)$$

Values of characteristic impedance of the aorta estimated from high frequency average of the input impedance spectrum have been variable, mostly due to the frequency range used for the estimation and the body size. In the dog, Z_o has been found to be 200-300 dyn.s.cm^5 when a typical high frequency range used for taking the average is 3-10 Hz. Higher frequency ranges can be used if significant harmonic magnitudes exist and are within measurement errors.

In the time domain, a simple method to approximate characteristic impedance of the aorta is to utilize the fact that in early ejection, peripheral reflected waves cannot reach the proximate aorta in appreciable amount over the time period. In this case, Z_o can be obtained relatively accurately, from the ratio of instantaneous aortic pressure, p(t) and flow Q(t) above their end-diastolic levels (Li, 1986):

$$Z_o = \frac{p(t) - p_d}{Q(t)} \qquad (4.2.10)$$

This method, as illustrated in Fig. 4.4.2, is valid for the first 60 ms of ejection when there is relative constancy of the instantaneous pressure to flow ratio (averaged over this time period). As noted earlier that this systolic ratio of pressure to flow (Li, 1991) can be influenced by reflections arising from local nonuniformities in geometry and elasticity

(Li *et al.*, 1984; Phan *et al.*, 2016). The time and frequency domain approaches to the estimation of Zo have been shown to correspond well (Li, 2000).

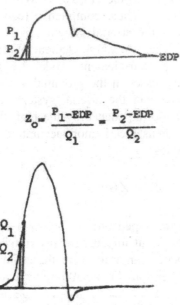

Fig. 4.2.2: Time-domain estimation of characteristic impedance (Zo) from early systolic phase of the aortic pressure and flow pulses. EDP=end-diastolic pressure.

Another method, also with the assumption that reflected waves do not significantly influence the measurement, is the classic water-hammer formula:

$$Z_o = \frac{\rho c}{\pi r^2} \tag{4.2.11}$$

where c is pulse wave velocity (PWV), r is radius and ρ is blood density, 1.06 g/cm^3. This method can be applied clinically where the cross-section area can be obtained with ultrasound echocardiograph and the foot-to-foot pulse wave velocity with dual-sensor catheter or Doppler ultrasound probes. More recently, phase contrast magnetic resonance imaging, or PC-MRI, has been used for noninvasive flow measurement and geometry for this purpose.

The relative contribution and the interplay of elastic properties and geometric factors to characteristic impedance have been analyzed for different arteries, in particular the brachial artery (Atlas and Li, 2003). Differences in vasoactive and mechanical loading can differentially alter aortic properties under isobaric conditions (Li *et al.*, 2010). The importance of smooth muscle activation has been shown to improve aortic compliance, hence its characteristic impedance during mechanical loading, as well demonstrated by Craim *et al.* (2011).

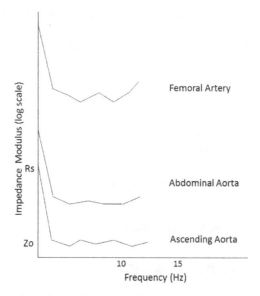

Fig. 4.2.3: Vascular impedances in the ascending aorta, abdominal aorta and the femoral artery showing increased impedance moduli away from the heart, with increased Rs and Zo values.

Both the input impedance and characteristic impedance moduli increase as the measurement site becomes further away from the heart, indicating greater impedance to blood flow. In addition, zero crossing of the phase occurs at a much higher frequency. Since only harmonic components can appear in the spectrum for a given heart rate, extended information can often be obtained by imposing cardiac pacing at different frequencies. The Vascular impedances obtained by Cox and Pace (1975) at aortic arch junction suffice to illustrate these. It is clear from those impedance spectra that ascending aorta has the lowest impedance modulus and the impedance modulus is higher through descending thoracic aorta, the left subclavian, the brachiocephalic and the carotid arteries. The characteristic impedances are also higher in smaller arteries due to their increased stiffness and reduced lumen diameter. Total peripheral resistance (mean or DC value at 0 Hz) of vascular beds that are perfused by smaller arteries is also higher.

Ventricular afterload is defined as all external factors that oppose ventricular ejection. For this reason arterial input impedance has been suggested as being the afterload. It is important to note that both the ability of the left ventricle to do work (myocardial performance) and the properties of the arterial system are important in determining the power generated by the ventricle.

In general, input impedance as predicted by the three-element Windkessel model gives a reasonable overall estimate of experimentally measured input impedance. This is more so in moduli than in phase. With vasoconstriction, the impedance modulus is increased and its first minimum is shifted to a higher frequency. With vasodilation, the impedance modulus decreases and its first minimum is shifted to a lower frequency. The corresponding zero-phase crossing also applies. This indicates that wave reflections arrive earlier due to a closer effective reflection site in the case of vasoconstriction.

4.3 Pulse Wave Propagation Phenomena

4.3.1 *The Pulse Wave Propagation Constant*

For a pressure pulse wave propagating along a uniform artery without the influence of wave reflections, the pressures measured simultaneously at any two sites along the vessel are related by:

$$p_2 = p_1 e^{-\gamma z} \tag{4.3.1}$$

where p_2 is the distal pressure, p_1 is the proximal pressure, γ is the propagation constant and z is along the longitudinal axis of the artery in the direction of pulse propagation. The propagation constant obtained under such circumstances, is known as the "true" propagation constant, since it is not influenced by wave reflections. It is a complex variable, thus has both magnitude and phase. It encompasses both the attenuation coefficient, α, and the phase constant, β:

$$\gamma = \alpha + j\beta \qquad (4.3.2)$$

The attenuation coefficient dictates the amount of damping imposed on the propagating pressure pulse due to both viscosity of the blood and viscosity of the arterial walls.

The phase constant arises because of the finite pulse wave velocity, c. In other words, the pressure pulse travels at finite velocity and therefore, takes finite amount of time to go through each arterial segment. Pulse wave velocity at any given frequency is given by:

$$c = \frac{\omega}{\beta} \qquad (4.3.3)$$

Thus, pulse wave velocity varies with frequency. This arises, because different harmonic component travels at different velocity, known as harmonic dispersion. Li *et al.* (1981) have shown that that true phase velocity increases at low frequencies and reach a somewhat constant value at high frequencies, usually beyond the third harmonic. Anliker *et al.* (1968) utilized high frequency artificial waves, essentially unaffected by reflections, to obtain phase velocity and attenuation in the dog aorta.

4.3.2 *Pulse Wave Velocity and the Foot-to-Foot Velocity*

Pulse wave velocity has been popularly approximated by the so-called "foot-to-foot" velocity. Here, one simply estimates the pulse wave velocity from the pulse transit time delay (PTT or Δt) of the "onset" or the "foot" between two pressure pulses measured at two different sites along an artery or the pulse propagation path. This requires again, the simultaneous measurements of two pressures separated by a finite distance, Δz, normally 4-6 cm apart. A double-lumen catheter with two pressure ports connected to two pressure transducers or a Millar catheter with dual pressure sensors suffice for such measurement. Thus, the foot-to-foot velocity, c_f is calculated from:

$$c_f = \frac{\Delta z}{\Delta t} \qquad (4.3.4)$$

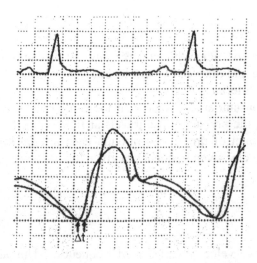

Fig. 4.3.1: Diagram illustrating how foot-to-foot velocity is calculated given pressure measurements at different sites separated by a known distance Δz. Here the foot-to-foot velocity is given by $c_f = \Delta z / \Delta t$. Δt is pulse transit time delay (PTT). Notice the peak-to-peak transit time is different from that of the foot-to-foot.

This method assumes that reflected waves do not interfere with the onset of the propagating pulse. As an example, referring to Fig. 4.3.1, the distance between the two pressure measurement sites is 5 cm and the calculated time delay, Δt, is 60 msec, or 0.06 sec, then the foot-to-foot velocity is

$$c_f = \frac{5}{0.06} = 833 \text{ cm/s} \qquad (4.3.5)$$

or 8.33 m/s.

Figure 4.3.2 shows the foot-to-foot velocity measured in different arteries (Nichols and McDonald, 1972). Wave velocity increased from about 5 m/s in the ascending aorta to about 10 m/s in the femoral artery, higher in the tibial artery.

Pulse wave velocity estimated from the peaks, or the peak-to-peak velocity, can give considerable errors, although the peak of the pulse is frequently easier to identify than the foot. This stems from the fact that the peak of the pressure pulse is often contaminated with reflected waves, since it allows sufficient time for reflected waves to arrive at the measurement sites.

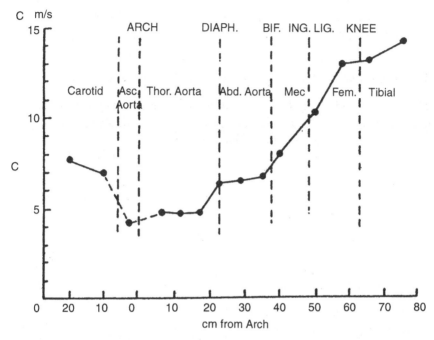

Fig. 4.3.2: Pulse wave velocity recorded as foot-to-foot velocity measured in different arteries. Higher wave velocities in smaller muscular arteries, such as the femoral and tibial, are seen. From Nichols and McDonald (1972).

With changing geometry and elastic properties away from the ascending aorta, the pulse wave velocity also changes. This is seen from the Moens-Korteweg formula for estimating pulse wave velocity:

$$c_o = \sqrt{\frac{Eh}{2\rho r}} \qquad (4.3.6)$$

where E is the elastic modulus of the artery, h and r are the wall thickness and radius of the artery and ρ is the density of blood. This formula is applicable to a single vessel, while foot-to-foot velocity has been obtained either for a single artery or over the pulse propagation path, e.g. over several arteries. Popular sites for noninvasive pulse wave velocity are brachial, radial, carotid and femoral arteries. For instance, carotid-to-femoral pulse wave velocity has been used as an index of vascular stiffness change in the aorta as is carotid-to-radial pulse wave velocity. It should be noted here pulse wave velocity measured over a long distance represents an "average" value, not specific of local arterial segment wall properties.

4.3.3 *Apparent Propagation Constant and Transfer Function*

There are considerable differences in the amount of wave reflections that arise in different parts of the circulation, owing to different vascular tree structure and neuro-humoral influences. In the presence of reflected waves, one can define an apparent propagation constant γ_{app} where

$$p_2 = p_1 e^{-\gamma_{app} z} \qquad (4.3.7)$$

$$\frac{p_2}{p_1} = e^{-\gamma_{app} z} \qquad (4.3.8)$$

and

$$\gamma_{app} = \frac{1}{\Delta z} \ln \frac{p_1}{p_2} \qquad (4.3.9)$$

The apparent propagation constant so defined is dependent on wave reflections and reflects local propagation characteristics. In this case, the separation (Δz) between p_2 and p_1 needs to be small, so that c_{app} is more representative of the underlying artery. When the separation is large, say from the ascending aorta to the abdominal aorta, the apparent wave velocity obtained may contain interactions resulting from branching vessels, with their vascular beds. On the other hand, the larger the distance of separation, gives much better accuracy or resolution of the attenuation and phase shift.

The apparent propagation constant at any point along the vessel is defined by:

$$\gamma_{app} = \alpha_{app} + j\beta_{app} \qquad (4.3.10)$$

and α_{app}, the apparent attenuation coefficient, is obtained from:

$$\alpha_{app} = \frac{1}{\Delta z} \ln \frac{|p_1|}{|p_2|} \qquad (4.3.11)$$

where $|p_1|$ and $|p_2|$ are the harmonic moduli of p_1 and p_2, respectively. It is clear that α_{app}, describes the degree of damping or the attenuation of the pressure pulse amplitude as it propagates between the two arterial sites.

The apparent phase constant β_{app} is obtained from:

$$\beta_{app} = (\phi_1 - \phi_2) / \Delta z \qquad (4.3.12)$$

where ϕ_1 and ϕ_2 are the harmonic phases of p_1 and p_2, respectively. The apparent phase velocity of propagation is calculated from:

$$c_{app} = \frac{\omega}{\beta_{app}} \qquad (4.3.13)$$

or more explicitly

$$c_{app} = \frac{2\pi f \cdot \Delta z}{\phi_1 - \phi_2} \qquad (4.3.14)$$

c_{app} is also known as the measured velocity. This apparent phase velocity is significantly affected by the presence of wave reflections, in the similar manner as vascular impedance.

The true and apparent propagation constants can be related to characteristic and input impedances as:

$$\frac{\gamma_{app}}{\gamma} = \frac{Z_o}{Z} \qquad (4.3.15)$$

This formula also provides a new method for obtaining true propagation constant from measured input impedance and apparent propagation constant (Li, 1987).

Because the apparent phase velocity, c_{app}, is influenced by wave reflections in the same manner that input impedance is affected, its frequency spectrum is similar to that of input impedance. Thus, γ_{app} is also influenced by wave reflections. An example of the frequency dependence of apparent propagation constant calculated for the femoral arterial bed is shown in Fig. 4.3.3. They are both dependent on the magnitude and phase of the global reflection coefficient (Γ). γ, on the other hand, is, by definition, independent of reflections, and the manner it varies with frequency has been quantified by Li *et al.* (1980, 1981). It can be deduced that, in the absence of reflected waves, $\Gamma=0$ and $\beta_{app}=\beta$, i.e., apparent phase velocity equals true phase velocity. This is easily seen from Fig. 4.3.4 from data obtained by Li *et al.* (1980) in a viscoelastic tube.

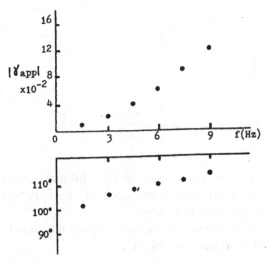

Fig. 4.3.3: Apparent propagation constant obtained as a function of frequency for the femoral arterial bed.

Apparent phase velocities have been obtained noninvasively with tonometers. One such example is shown in Fig. 4.3.5. The pressure waveforms were first obtained and the apparent phase velocity spectra calculated between the carotid and radial arterial sites for normal and hypertensive adults (Li *et al.*, 1996). It must be stated that estimation of c_{app} over a long propagation path usually subject to more random summation and cancellation of reflected waves within the path.

The definition of apparent propagation constant, γ_{app}, by eqn. (4.3.9) also represents what is popularly known as the "pressure transfer function", or simply transfer function. Thus, knowing the transfer function of two arterial sites, one can obtain one blood pressure waveform from the other. This follows from the definition of apparent propagation constant (eqns. (4.3.7) and (4.3.9)). For, instant, one can obtain the central aortic pressure waveform from carotid pressure pulse measurement, if the apparent propagation constant or the transfer function is known. Since carotid pulse, radial pulse and brachial pulse can be readily obtained noninvasively, this transfer function method has attracted clinical interest in recent years. The goal is to obtain central aortic pressure from noninvasive peripheral arterial pulse measurement.

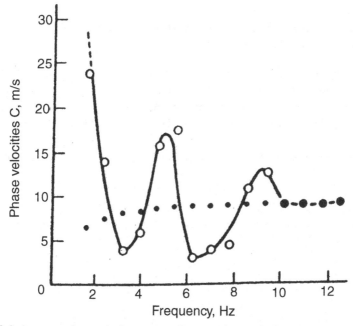

Fig. 4.3.4: Apparent phase velocity compared to true phase velocity in a viscoelastic tube. The influence of wave reflections on apparent phase velocity at low frequencies is clearly seen. At high frequencies the two velocities approach a somewhat constant value that is approximated by the foot-to-foot pulse wave velocity.

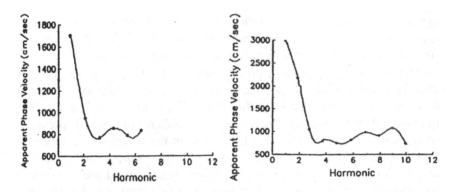

Fig. 4.3.5: Apparent phase velocities obtained by noninvasive pressure measurements with tonometers at the carotid and radial arterial sites in normal and hypertensive adults. Larger low frequency amplitudes and greater oscillations at higher frequencies can be seen.

4.3.4 *Determination of the Propagation Constant and Frequency Dependent Pulse Wave Velocity*

Experimental determination of the apparent propagation constant is simpler than that of the true propagation constant. The former can be determined by simultaneously measuring either two pressures for the pressure pulse, or two flows for the flow pulse. Determination of the true propagation constant which is independent of wave reflections, in the presence of reflections, however, requires simultaneous measurement of three variables.

Several methods are available to determine the true propagation constant, all of which are based on linear transmission line theory. From the definition of the propagation constant as it relates to longitudinal (Z_l) and transverse (Z_t) impedances:

$$\gamma = \sqrt{Z_l / Z_t} \qquad (4.3.16)$$

where

$$Z_l = \frac{-\partial p / \partial z}{Q} \qquad (4.3.17)$$

$$Z_t = \frac{-p}{\partial Q / \partial z} \qquad (4.3.18)$$

Knowing these relationships, the measurement of pressure and flow together with their gradients permit determination of the propagation constant. Thus, one can apply this method by measuring two pressures and two flows, or by measuring two pressures, a few centimeters apart, a flow midway between them, and the pulsatile change in diameter. Alternatively, the transverse impedance, which is related to vessel wall properties, can be obtained from the dynamic pressure-area relationship. If two pressures and flows are measured simultaneously at two sites along a uniform vessel, the propagation constant can be obtained from:

$$\gamma = \frac{1}{\Delta z} \cosh^{-1} [\frac{p_1 Q_1 + p_2 Q_2}{p_2 Q_1 + p_1 Q_2}] \qquad (4.3.19)$$

where Δz denotes the distance between the two sites. Subscript $_1$ refers to the upstream site and $_2$, the downstream site.

Another method utilizes the simultaneous recording of three pressures along a uniform vessel. The propagation constant is obtained as:

$$\gamma = \frac{1}{\Delta z} \cosh^{-1} [\frac{\Delta p_1 + \Delta p_3}{2 p_2}] \qquad (4.3.20)$$

when differential pressures are measured, $\Delta p_1 = p_1 - p_2$; $\Delta p_3 = p_3 - p_2$. The three pressures p_1, p_2, p_3, are simultaneously measured at an equal distance (Δz) apart.

The three-point pressure method was extensively evaluated by Li *et al.* (1980) in a hydrodynamic model. Subsequently, this method was applied to investigate pulse wave propagation in dogs (Li *et al.*, 1981) with respect to contributions by vascular wall elastic and geometric properties, vessel wall and blood viscosity, and nonlinearities in system parameters and in the equations of motion. Discrepancies in results obtained with different experimental methods and theory were discussed and resolved. Measurements were obtained from the abdominal aorta, as well as the carotid, iliac, and femoral arteries of dogs. The components of the propagation constant, i.e., attenuation coefficient and phase velocity, were obtained for each of the vessels investigated (Figures 4.3.6 and 4.3.7).

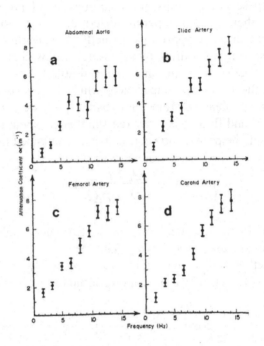

Fig. 4.3.6: Attenuation coefficients obtained for the lower abdominal aorta (a), iliac artery (b), femoral artery (c), and carotid artery (d). Greater attenuation, hence damping of the propagating pulse wave is seen in muscular arteries, such as the femoral artery, compared with the elastic aorta. Mean±SEM.

Results were presented along a continuous path of transmission (abdominal aorta, iliac, femoral) and it was shown that variations in phase velocity can be explained entirely by the geometric and elastic variation of these vessels. Phase velocities were shown to be frequency independent at > 4 Hz, while attenuation increases progressively for higher frequencies. The three-point method was also applied by Wells *et al.* (1998) to infer the contributions of collagen and elastin to overall viscoelastic properties of sheep thoracic aorta.

In terms of attenuation, it is clear that blood pressure pulse is more damped while propagating away from the heart. This is seen when comparing the attenuation coefficient of abdominal aorta with that of the femoral artery (Fig. 4.3.6). The amount of damping increases with frequency, indicating that higher frequency components, such as the dicrotic notch prominent in the central aorta, becoming rounded in the femoral artery pressure waveform (see Fig. 4.1.2).

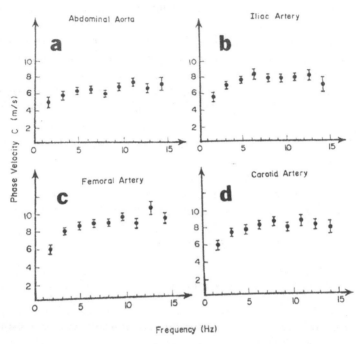

Fig. 4.3.7: Phase velocities obtained in the (a) lower abdominal aorta, (b) iliac artery, (c) femoral artery, and (d) carotid artery.

Increased wall thickness-to-radius ratio (h/r) in muscular arteries (e.g. femoral) and higher elastic modulus, both contribute to higher pulse wave velocity. This is seen in Fig. 4.3.7 where femoral arterial phase velocity is significantly higher than abdominal aorta. Pulse wave velocity based on commonly measured foot-to-foot velocity approximates the high frequency average of the frequency dependent phase velocity. At higher frequencies (higher harmonic components of the pulse wave), phase velocity is relatively constant.

4.4 Pulse Wave Reflection Phenomena

4.4.1 *Influence of Wave Reflections on Pressure and Flow Waveforms*

The amplification of pressure pulses has been attributed to the in-phase summation of reflected waves arising from structural and geometric nonuniformities. The microvascular beds have been recognized as the principal reflection sites. Thus, pulsatile pressure and flow waveforms contain information about the heart as well as the vascular system. Reflection in the vascular system has been suggested as a closed-end type, as pressure is amplified and flow diminishes, with arterioles being the major reflection site. By definition, reflected pressure and flow waves are 180° out of phase. This means an increase in reflection increases pulse pressure amplitude, but decreases pulsatile flow amplitude.

Pressure (P) and flow (Q) waveforms measured at any site in the vascular system can be considered as the summation of a forward, or antegrade, traveling wave and a reflected, or retrograde, traveling wave:

$$P = P_f + P_r \qquad\qquad (4.4.1)$$

$$Q = Q_f + Q_r \qquad\qquad (4.4.2)$$

The forward and reflected pressure components can be resolved by means of the following set of equations:

$$P_f = (P + Q \cdot Zo) / 2 \qquad\qquad (4.4.3)$$

$$P_r = (P - Q \cdot Zo) / 2 \qquad\qquad (4.4.4)$$

where Z_0 is the characteristic impedance, defined as the ratio of forward pressure to forward flow, or in other words, independent of wave reflections:

$$Z_o = \frac{P_f}{Q_f} = -\frac{P_r}{Q_r} \qquad\qquad (4.4.5)$$

Z_o can be obtained from the water-hammer formula, shown previously,

$$Z_o = \frac{\rho c}{\pi r^2} \qquad (4.4.6)$$

where ρ is the density of blood (1.06 g/cm^3), c is pulse wave velocity, πr^2 is the cross-sectional area of the artery. With the characteristic impedance determined by a time domain method, forward and reflected waves can also be resolved in the time domain (Li, 1986). This approach is known as the time-domain wave separation method, which has been widely used.

Similarly, resolution of flow into its forward and reflected components can be obtained from a set of two equations:

$$Q_f = (Q + P / Z_o) / 2 \qquad (4.4.7)$$

$$Q_r = (Q - P / Z_o) / 2 \qquad (4.4.8)$$

From the above equations, it can be seen that wave reflection has opposite effects on pressure and flow. An increase in wave reflection increases the pressure amplitude, but decreases the flow amplitude. This is particularly evident during different spontaneous or induced vasoactive states. Figure 4.4.1 illustrates the pressure and flow waveforms recorded during control, vasoconstriction and vasodilation conditions. Vasoconstriction is induced by intravenous infusion of methoxamine (MTX), a potent vasoconstrictor. Its primary effect is in increasing peripheral vascular resistance and has little cardiac effect. Vasodilation is induced by intravenous infusion of nitroprusside (NTP). This is a common vasodilator that can profoundly decrease peripheral vascular resistance and increase arterial compliance. It can be seen that the pressure waveform during strong vasodilation more closely resembles that of the flow waveform. Other popularly used vasoactive drugs are phenylephrine and nitroglycerine for inducing vasoconstriction and vasodilation, respectively.

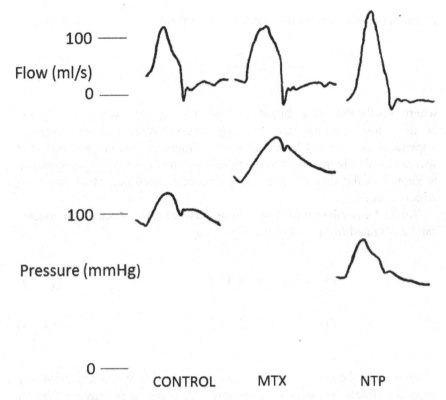

Fig. 4.4.1: Simultaneously recorded ascending aortic pressure and flow waveforms during control (left), methoxamine (MTX) induced vasoconstriction (middle) and nitroprusside (NTP) induced vasodilation (right).

Aortic pressure (top) and flow (bottom) waveforms resolved into their respective forward (Pf, Qf) or antegrade, and reflected (Pr, Qr) or retrograde components are shown in Fig. 4.4.2. It is clear that wave reflection exerts opposite effects on pressure and flow waveforms. The increased reflected pressure component adds to the forward wave to result in the measured pressure waveform. Reflected wave has a more significant effect in mid- to late systole to impede ventricular ejection. Wave reflection decreases the flow, as the reflected component of flow is mostly negative.

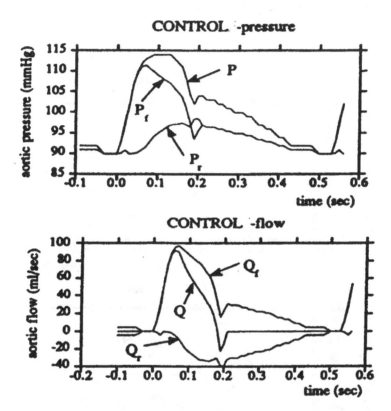

Fig. 4.4.2: Ascending aortic pressure (top) and flow (bottom) waveforms resolved into their respective forward (P_f, Q_f) or antegrade, and reflected (P_r, Q_r) or retrograde components. Notice that wave reflection exerts opposite effects on pressure and flow waveforms, as seen from Q_r and P_r. Provided by Dr. Janet Ying Zhu.

With an increased amount of wave reflection, the pressure amplitude is increased. This is seen in the case of strong vasoconstriction shown in Fig. 4.4.3. Here reflected waves arrive earlier and with greater magnitudes. As a consequence, the pulse pressure is significantly increased with a concurrent decrease in flow amplitude. The time that takes for forward pressure to reach its peak is not too different from that of the reflected component. With profound vasodilation (Fig. 4.4.4), the measured pressure and flow waveforms resemble each other and both peak at about the same time. The reflected wave is largely abolished. Thus, both pressure and flow waves are transmitted with maximal efficiency.

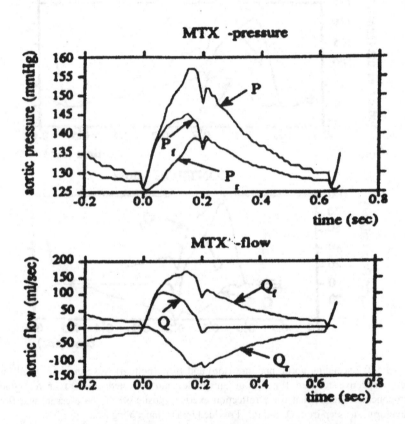

Fig. 4.4.3: Ascending aortic pressure and flow waveforms resolved into their respective forward and reflected components during vasoconstriction induced by intravenous infusion of methoxamine. Notice the significantly increased reflected pressure component. Provided by Dr. Janet Ying Zhu.

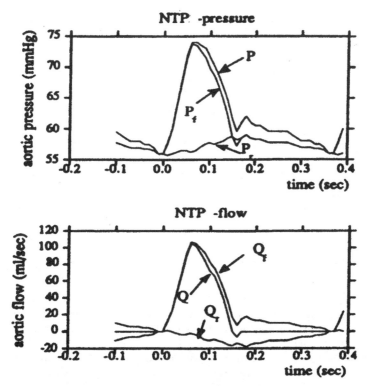

Fig. 4.4.4: Ascending aortic pressure and flow waveforms resolved into their respective forward and reflected components during vasodilation induced by intravenous infusion of nitroprusside. Notice the similarity between the pressure and flow waveforms and that the reflected components are small. Provided by Dr. Janet Ying Zhu.

Pulse pressure amplitude alone often does not indicate the underlying factors governing the morphology of blood pressure pulse waveforms, although its increase has been shown to correlate with an increase in vascular stiffness. Thus, the routine clinically used cuff method for measuring systolic and diastolic pressures cannot be used to infer contributing factors to vascular stiffness or arterial properties. One example is shown in Fig. 4.4.5 that despite similar systolic and diastolic pressures induced either by change in mechanical properties of the blood vessel wall or change in vasoactive states, the forward and reflected waveform morphologies and contributing factors differ (Li *et al.*, 2010). A wave reflection-based distributed model (Zhang and Li, 2009) can be used to resolve the vasoactive from mechanical factors.

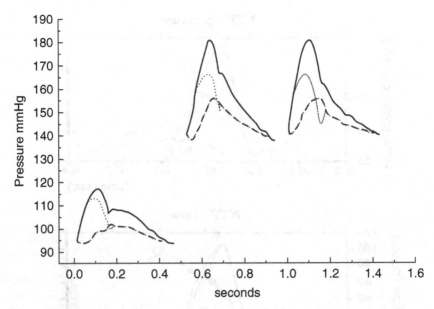

Fig. 4.4.5: Ascending aortic pressure and flow waveforms resolved into their respective forward and reflected components during control (left), descending thoracic aorta occlusion (center) and methoxamine induced hypertension (right). Although pulse pressures are about the same due to mechanical (DTA) or vasoactive (MTX) interventions, the underlying morphology and forward and reflected waves differ.

4.4.2 *The Reflection Coefficients*

The reflection coefficient is defined as the harmonic ratio of reflected wave to the forward wave in the frequency domain:

$$\Gamma = \frac{P_r}{P_f} \qquad (4.4.9)$$

It has both a modulus and a phase, and varies with frequency:

$$\Gamma = |\Gamma| \angle \phi_\Gamma \qquad (4.4.10)$$

Reflection coefficients calculated for the normal, vasoconstricted and vasodilated conditions obtained from canine experiments are shown in Fig. 4.4.6. For the fundamental harmonic, the mean value of the reflection coefficient at control is about 0.45. This is increased to 0.65 during vasoconstriction and decreased to about 0.15 during vasodilation. The reflection coefficient remains low for higher frequencies during vasodilation.

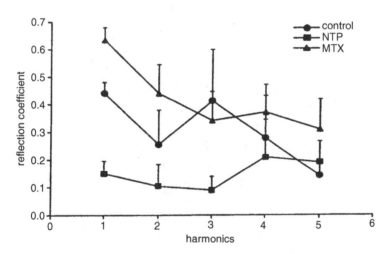

Fig. 4.4.6: Global reflection coefficients (Γ) obtained during control (circle), vasoconstriction (triangle) and vasodilation (square) conditions.

Reflection coefficient can also be defined in terms of vascular impedances. For a vessel with characteristic impedance Z_o and terminated with vascular load impedance Z, the reflection coefficient Γ is given by:

$$\Gamma = \frac{Z - Z_o}{Z + Z_o} \qquad (4.4.11)$$

The reflection coefficient so obtained is therefore a complex quantity with modulus Γ and phase ϕ_Γ varying with frequency, as before. Thus, the magnitude and timing of arrival of reflected waves are both important in modifying the propagating pulse. Comparison of time and frequency domain descriptions of the reflection coefficients have been provided by Lei *et al.* (1996). Additionally, the global reflection coefficient presented here is in general, masked by the repeated reflections (Berger *et al.*, 1993) from multiple reflection sites in the arterial system. These latter are important considerations.

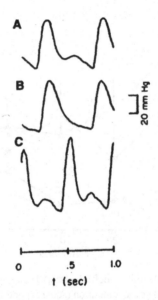

Fig. 4.4.7: Pressure waveforms measured in the femoral artery during control (A), acetylcholine induced vasodilated (B), and norepinephrine induced vasoconstricted (C) states. Notice the diastolic wave is significantly augmented in vasoconstriction and abolished in vasodilation.

The reflection coefficient can also be defined for a particular vascular bed. For instance, Li *et al.* (1984) utilized a three-point pressure method to measure the amount of reflections arising from the femoral arterial bed during (a) control, (b) acetylcholine-induced vasodilation, and (c) norepinephrine-induced vasoconstriction states (Fig. 4.4.7). Notice that the diastolic pressure wave is abolished during acetylcholine-induced vasodilation and accentuated during norepinephrine-induced vasoconstriction.

Computed reflection coefficients obtained for the femoral vascular bed are shown in Fig. 4.4.8. For the control data (circle), the magnitude of the reflection coefficient ranged from 0.42 at 1.6 Hz, to 0.22 at 9.6 Hz. During vasoconstriction, the reflection coefficient increased to about 0.65 at 1.6 Hz and 0.32 at 9.6 Hz. Vasodilation (triangles) decreased the reflection coefficient to a value less than 0.1 for all frequencies, essentially abolishing the reflected waves. This is clear from Fig. 4.4.6.

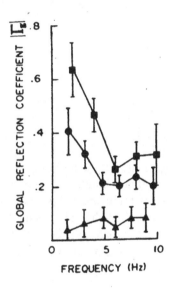

Fig. 4.4.8: Reflections arising from the femoral vascular bed during control (circle), vasoconstriction (square) and vasodilation (triangle). Reflection coefficients were computed from the three-point method.

4.4.3 The Augmentation Index

Since large vessel properties can appreciably affect ventricular ejection, aortic compliance and wave reflections appearing in the aorta have become important markers for assessing arterial system behavior in the clinical setting. Since frequency domain interpretation of wave reflections is complex and cumbersome to obtain, a simplified index to interpret wave reflection in the aorta, in the time domain, was introduced by Murgo *et al.* (1980). Ascending aortic pressure waveforms were defined in terms of their morphological differences and separated into different types. Peak systolic pressure (P_s or P_{pk}), diastolic pressure (P_d), pulse pressure (PP), pressure at inflection point (P_i) where peak flow occurs, and the augmented pressure, ΔP are defined. Systolic pressure augmentation is given by

$$\Delta P = P_s - P_i \qquad (4.4.12)$$

and the corresponding augmentation index (AIx) for the aorta is given by

$$AIx = \frac{\Delta P}{PP} = \frac{P_s - P_i}{P_s - P_d} \qquad (4.4.13)$$

Although simple to compute and widely used in the clinical setting to infer the amount of wave reflections or to represent the reflection ratio, it is not equivalent to the reflection coefficient. Augmentation index is merely a single number and cannot represent the frequency content of the reflected wave, its timing of arrival or temporal amplitude. In addition, the inflection pressure is often obtained at the early upstroke of the systolic aortic pressure when there are supposedly less reflected waves present. As we have seen earlier that significantly greater amount of reflected waves occurs in mid- to late systole (e.g. Fig. 4.4.2). Thus, AIx in general underestimates the amount of wave reflections. This is clear when comparing AIx with the fundamental (first harmonic) reflection coefficient.

Another index based on the peripheral pressure pulse, typically radial arterial pulse, has been proposed as the peripheral augmentation index (AIXp; Millasseau *et al.*, 2003). While radial artery based AIXp has shown to be correlated to transfer function synthesized aortic AIx, it can be significantly affected by local vasoactive conditions which may not directly affect central aorta or large vessel compliance, hence aortic augmentation index.

4.4.4 *Wave Reflection Sites and Multiple Reflections*

Wave reflection sites exist all over the systemic arterial tree, due to geometric and elastic nonuniformities, branching, and impedance mismatching at arterial terminations, in addition to rapidly changing vasoactive states and neuro-humoral influences. Therefore, pulse wave reflections do not originate from a single site. Indeed, there is no agreement on the location of reflecting sites. Some suggest that the major reflection site as seen from the proximal aorta, appears to be in the region of the pelvis or the aorto-iliac branching junction. Others, however, suggest that the first major potential reflecting site is at the aortic arch. Although there is no major agreement on the reflecting sites, the arterioles are recognized as being the principal sites for wave reflection, and the reflection coefficient as being high.

There are multiple reflection sites and the effects of repeated reflections on pressure and flow waveforms have been investigated (Berger *et al.*, 1993). The model-based analysis showed how the forward and reflected waves are actually the summations of repeated antegrade and retrograde waves. The dispersion of such multiple reflections makes direct measurement and quantification of their individual contributions to global reflection phenomenon a demanding task.

Reflection sites have generally been determined from the first impedance minimum, and subsequent calculation, based on the quarter-wavelength concept from linear transmission line theory:

$$\lambda_{min} = \frac{c}{f_{min}} \qquad (4.4.14)$$

and

$$L_R = \frac{\lambda_{min}}{4} \qquad (4.4.15)$$

λ_{min} and f_{min} are the wavelength and frequency corresponding to the impedance minimum. L_R is the distance of the effective reflection site from the point of measurement. Some investigators have used the zero-phase crossing of impedance for the calculation of effective reflection sites. This makes assumption of the impedance of the vascular terminations critical in the interpretation of the amount of wave reflections.

4.5 Modeling Aspects of the Arterial Circulation

4.5.1 *Mathematical Formulations of Pulse Wave Propagation*

There are three equations generally thought to be sufficient to characterize the propagation of the pulse wave. The first of these equations describes fluid motion,

$$-\frac{\partial v_z}{\partial t} = \frac{1}{\rho}\frac{\partial p}{\partial z} \tag{4.5.1}$$

where v_z is the blood velocity in the longitudinal z direction or along the blood vessel from proximal to distal locations, p is pressure and ρ is the density of blood. The left side of the equation represents the rate of change of velocity, or flow acceleration. This equation implies that blood flow acceleration is proportional to the pressure gradient. For this reason, this formula has been used to obtain blood flow from the measurement of pressure gradient. This latter is obtained by the simultaneous measurements of two pressures at known distance apart.

The second is the equation of continuity to describe the incompressibility of the fluid:

$$-\frac{\partial v_z}{\partial z} = \frac{1}{A}\frac{\partial A}{\partial t} = \frac{2}{r}\frac{\partial r}{\partial t} \tag{4.5.2}$$

or that blood flow velocity gradient is related to the rate of change in cross-sectional area of the blood vessel. In a cylindrical blood vessel the cross-sectional area A is related to its inner lumen radius r, as $A=\pi r^2$.

The third equation is the equation of state to describe the elastic properties of the vessel wall

$$\frac{dr}{dp} = k \tag{4.5.3}$$

where k is a constant.

From this set of three equations encompassing the fluid-wall interaction, the well-known wave equation is obtained as:

$$\frac{\partial^2 v_z}{\partial t^2} = \frac{r}{2k\rho} \frac{\partial^2 v_z}{\partial z^2} \qquad (4.5.4)$$

which gives the wave velocity

$$c_o = (\frac{r}{2k\rho})^{\frac{1}{2}} = (\frac{r}{2\rho} \frac{dp}{dr})^{\frac{1}{2}} \qquad (4.5.5)$$

This equation also provides a means to obtain pulse wave velocity from the simultaneous measurements of pressure and diameter. Define Young's modulus of elasticity as stress over strain:

$$E = \frac{\sigma_t}{\varepsilon_t} \qquad (4.5.6)$$

Using the Lame equation for stress

$$\sigma_t = \frac{pr}{h} \qquad (4.5.7)$$

and write radial strain as

$$\varepsilon_t = \frac{dr}{r} \qquad (4.5.8)$$

We obtain a similar wave equation:

$$\frac{\partial^2 v_z}{\partial t^2} = \frac{Eh}{2r\rho} \frac{\partial^2 v_z}{\partial z^2} \qquad (4.5.9)$$

which gives the pulse wave velocity as:

$$c_o = \sqrt{\frac{Eh}{2\rho r}} \qquad (4.5.10)$$

This is the well-known Moens-Korteweg formula for pulse wave velocity (Li, 1987, 2000). Moens in 1878 obtained this formula through experimentation and obtained

$$c_o = k_m \sqrt{\frac{Eh}{2\rho r}} \qquad (4.5.11)$$

where k_m is a constant. Korteweg, also at about the same time, approached from a theoretical perspective by assuming a flat velocity profile, ignoring viscosity and fluid compressibility, and imposing vessel wall constraints and obtained an identical formula (Noordergraaf, 1969; Li, 1987).

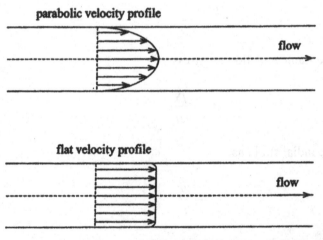

Fig. 4.5.1: Velocity profiles in different arteries. A blunt or flat velocity profile (bottom tracing) is when the blood velocity across the vessel is uniform, mostly find in large vessels, such as the proximal aorta. A parabolic velocity profile (top tracing) is when the centerline velocity is the highest with decreasing velocity towards the arterial wall, occurring when velocity is fully developed. A skewed velocity profile is when the blood velocity is high towards one wall than the opposite side.

The flat velocity profile implies that the blood flow velocity across the artery is uniform. In a parabolic velocity profile, the centerline velocity is the highest and the velocity declines in a parabolic fashion towards the vessel wall, such that at the arterial wall, the velocity is the lowest

(Fig. 4.5.1). In the arterial system, the velocity profile is relatively flat or blunt at the entrance, or at the ascending aorta and becomes progressively parabolic when approaching smaller arteries.

Lamb (1898) later assumed an inviscid, or non-viscous, fluid contained within a thin-walled tube (h<<r) subject to small strains and arrived at equations of motion for the wall:

$$\rho_w \frac{\partial^2 u_z}{\partial t^2} = \frac{E}{1-\sigma^2}\left(\frac{\partial^2 u_z}{\partial z^2} + \frac{\sigma}{r}\frac{\partial u_z}{\partial z}\right) \qquad (4.5.12)$$

$$\rho_w \frac{\partial^2 u_r}{\partial t^2} = \frac{p}{h}\frac{E}{1-\sigma^2}\left(\frac{\sigma}{r}\frac{\partial u_z}{\partial z} + \frac{u_r}{r^2}\right) \qquad (4.5.13)$$

Where u_z and u_r are wall movement in the longitudinal and radial directions respectively. These equations were later incorporated by many investigators in the analysis of pulse wave propagation and fluid-wall interaction. Lamb obtained two roots for the wave velocity from a quadratic equation he derived. One is identical to the Moens-Korteweg formula, or Young's mode velocity of propagation, with the propagation wavelength much greater than the vessel lumen radius, or $\lambda >> r$ and Poisson ratio $\sigma = 0.5$, describing the incompressibility of fluid:

$$c_1 = \sqrt{\frac{Eh}{2\rho r}} \qquad (4.5.14)$$

The other is now known as the Lamb mode velocity for wave propagating longitudinally in the arterial wall:

$$c_1 = \sqrt{\frac{Eh}{\rho(1-\sigma^2)}} \qquad (4.5.15)$$

Velocities given in the longitudinal and radial directions are given by:

$$v_z = \left[C_2 \frac{J_0(jr\sqrt{j\omega\rho/\eta}}{J_0(jr_i\sqrt{j\omega\rho/\eta}} + \frac{A_2}{\rho c} \right] e^{j\omega(t-z/c)} \qquad (4.5.16)$$

$$v_r = \left[\frac{\omega}{c}\sqrt{\frac{\eta}{j\omega\rho}} C_2 \frac{J_1(jr\sqrt{j\omega\rho/\eta}}{J_0(jr_i\sqrt{j\omega\rho/\eta}} + \frac{j\omega r}{2\rho c^2} A \right] e^{j\omega(t-z/c)} \qquad (4.5.17)$$

where J_0 and J_1 are zero and first order Bessel functions of the first kind.

4.5.2 *Linear Theories of Oscillatory Blood Flow in Arteries*

In general, linear theories regarding blood flow begin with the fundamental Navier-Stokes equations for a Newtonian and incompressible fluid (Attinger, 1964) in cylindrical coordinates, and assuming irrotational flow. Pulsatile pressure and flow relations, as well as complex velocity of wave propagation can be obtained (Li, 1987).

Navier-Stokes equations for a Newtonian and incompressible fluid in cylindrical coordinates (r, θ, z) and assuming irrotational flow, i.e. the angular θ components are negligible, can be written as:

$$\frac{\partial v_z}{\partial t} + v_r \frac{\partial v_z}{\partial r} + v_z \frac{\partial v_z}{\partial z} = -\frac{1}{\rho}\frac{\partial p}{\partial z} + \frac{\eta}{\rho}\left(\frac{\partial^2 v_z}{\partial r^2} + \frac{1}{r}\frac{\partial v_z}{\partial r} + \frac{\partial^2 v_z}{\partial z^2} \right)$$

$$\frac{\partial v_r}{\partial t} + v_r \frac{\partial v_r}{\partial r} + v_z \frac{\partial v_r}{\partial z} = -\frac{1}{\rho}\frac{\partial p}{\partial z} + \frac{\eta}{\rho}\left(\frac{\partial^2 v_r}{\partial r^2} + \frac{1}{r}\frac{\partial v_r}{\partial r} + \frac{\partial^2 v_r}{\partial z^2} - \frac{v_r}{r^2} \right)$$

$$(4.5.18)$$

where v_z = longitudinal velocity component
v_r = radial velocity component
η = viscosity of blood
and η/ρ = kinematic viscosity of blood

Notice that when the fluid is assumed to be ideal, i.e. kinematic viscosity $\eta/\rho = 0$, the equations reduce to:

$$\frac{1}{r}\frac{\partial}{\partial r}(rv_r) = -\frac{\partial v_z}{\partial z} \tag{4.5.19}$$

For linearized Navier-Stokes equations, the second and third terms of the left-hand side of (4.5.18) are negligible for small velocities. For long wavelength ($\lambda \gg r$), or Young's mode, one obtains solutions as follows, for a periodic sinusoidal varying function $e^{j\omega(t-z/c)}$ of pressure:

$$p = -A\omega\rho e^{j\omega(t-z/c)} \tag{4.5.20}$$

$$v_z = \left[-\frac{A_1\omega}{c} + C_1\sqrt{\frac{j\omega\rho}{\eta}} J_0\left(jr\sqrt{\frac{j\omega\rho}{\eta}}\right) \right] e^{j\omega(t-z/c)} \tag{4.5.21}$$

$$v_r = -\left[\frac{jA_1\omega^2 r}{2c^2} - \frac{C_1\omega}{c} J_1\left(jr\sqrt{\frac{j\omega\rho}{\eta}}\right) \right] e^{j\omega(t-z/c)} \tag{4.5.22}$$

where J_0 and J_1 are the zero and first order Bessel functions of the first kind, and A_1 and C_1 are constants.

By using Lamb's equations for the wall and applying the boundary condition that fluid and wall velocities are equal at the wall, i.e.

$$v_z(r = r_i) = \frac{\partial u_z}{\partial t} \tag{4.5.23}$$

and

$$v_r(r = r_i) = \frac{\partial u_r}{\partial t} \tag{4.5.24}$$

a complex velocity of propagation is obtained as

$$c_1 = k\sqrt{\frac{Eh}{2\rho r}} \tag{4.5.25}$$

where k contains Bessel functions J_0 and J_1. For k = 1, as in the case when the fluid is ideal, i.e. the kinematic viscosity $\eta/\rho = 0$, this equation reduces to the familiar Moens-Korteweg formula for pulse wave velocity.

Differences in linearized theories are mostly in the description of arterial wall properties and arterial wall motion. More accurate descriptions of the blood-arterial wall interactions can be achieved by additions or improvements in the equations describing the wall and blood, or the so-called blood-wall interactions. These latter arise because of the fluid-tissue interface and the differences in mechanical behaviors. Indeed, modern clinical analysis has placed more emphasis on the blood-endothelial interface and on the blood flow and elastin-collagen interactions, as well as smooth muscle activation.

Morgan and Kiely (1954) added viscous fluid stress terms to the Lamb eqns. (4.5.12 and 4.5.13):

$$-\frac{\eta}{h}(\frac{\partial v_z}{\partial r} + \frac{\partial v_r}{\partial z})_{r=r_i} \qquad (4.5.26)$$

$$-\frac{2\eta}{h}(\frac{\partial v_z}{\partial r})_{r=r_i} \qquad (4.5.27)$$

a parameter, now known as the Womersley's parameter was introduced:

$$\alpha_w = r\sqrt{\frac{\omega\rho}{\eta}} \qquad (4.5.28)$$

$$\omega = 2\pi f_h \qquad (4.5.29)$$

$$f_h = \text{heart rate/sec} \qquad (4.5.30)$$

ρ (1.06 g/cm^3) and η (0.03 poise or 3 centipoise) are the density and viscosity of blood, respectively and r is the inner radius of the artery. This Womersley's parameter also represents the ratio of the relative contribution of inertia component to viscous component of blood flow. In other words, it describes the ratio of the movement of blood mass to the retardation of flow or flow resistance due to blood viscosity. α_ω is also dependent on arterial lumen radius, thus, the smaller the vessel, the smaller the value of α_ω.

Morgan and Kiely made assumptions to arrive at wave velocity and damping coefficient (α), for $r = r_i$ and $\alpha_\omega \gg 1$:

$$c = \left[1 - \frac{1}{r}(1 - \sigma + \frac{\sigma^2}{4})(\frac{\eta}{2\omega\rho})^{\frac{1}{2}} \right] \sqrt{\frac{Eh}{2r\rho}} \qquad (4.5.31)$$

And for for $\alpha_\omega \ll 1$

$$\alpha = \frac{\omega}{r} \left[\frac{\eta(5 - 4\sigma)}{\omega\rho} \right]^{\frac{1}{2}} \sqrt{\frac{2r\rho}{Eh}} \qquad (4.5.32)$$

For extremely low frequencies, or in the case of very small vessels, these equations can be compared to those derived earlier.

Many linear theories of oscillating blood flow in arteries have been proposed, but that of Womersley's remains the most commonly used. A frequency dependent parameter not originally defined by him, but later known as the Womersley's parameter was introduced, as shown in eqn. (4.5.28). Womersley (1957) also utilized a linearized Navier-Stokes equation, and an equation of motion of a freely moving elastic tube with homogeneous and isotropic wall material. He also made assumptions that the pulse propagation wavelength is much greater than that of the arterial lumen radius, or $\lambda \gg r$, and that the propagating pressure pulse takes the form of

$$p = A\, e^{j\omega(t-z/c)} \qquad (4.5.33)$$

where A is the amplitude of the pressure pulse (p) and c is pulse wave velocity. He obtained

$$v_z = \left[C_2 \frac{J_0(jr\sqrt{j\omega\rho/\eta})}{J_0(jr_i\sqrt{j\omega\rho/\eta})} + \frac{A_2}{\rho c} \right] e^{j\omega(t-z/c)} \qquad (4.5.34)$$

$$v_r = \left[\frac{\omega}{c}\sqrt{\frac{\eta}{j\omega\rho}} C_2 \frac{J_1(jr\sqrt{j\omega\rho/\eta})}{J_0(jr_i\sqrt{j\omega\rho/\eta})} + \frac{j\omega r}{2\rho c^2} A \right] e^{j\omega(t-z/c)} \qquad (4.5.35)$$

An equation for the pulse wave velocity was derived, assuming arterial wall and blood densities are equal,

$$c = \sqrt{\frac{r\rho}{hE}} k_c \qquad (4.5.36)$$

where k_c is a function of the Bessel function

$$F_{10} = \frac{2J_1(\alpha j^{3/2})}{\alpha j^{3/2} J_0(\alpha j^{3/2})} \qquad (4.5.37)$$

Where again J_0 and J_1, are zero and first order Bessel functions of the first kind. Solutions for J_0 and J_1, are tabulated by Womersley and van Brummelen (1961). Rewrite F_{10} in its complex form in terms of real and imaginary parts, we have:

$$F_{10} = X + jY \qquad (4.5.38)$$

Womersley obtained an expression for complex wave velocity:

$$c = \frac{1}{X - jY} \sqrt{\frac{Eh}{2r\rho}} \qquad (4.5.39)$$

From this, the phase velocity is:

$$c_1 = \frac{c_o}{X} \qquad X = \frac{c_1}{c_o} \qquad (4.5.40)$$

noting again that the Moens-Korteweg wave velocity is given by

$$c_o = \sqrt{\frac{Eh}{2r\rho}} \qquad (4.5.41)$$

The attenuation expressed in terms of wavelength is given by:

$$\alpha_e = e^{-2\pi Y/X\lambda} \qquad (4.5.42)$$

Attenuation represents the degree of damping of the propagating pulse.

Womersley later imposed longitudinal constraint of the wall due to vessel tethering. In the case of infinite longitudinal constraint, k_∞, wave velocity takes the form:

$$\frac{c_o}{c} = \sqrt{\frac{1-\sigma^2}{1-F_{10}}} \qquad (4.5.43)$$

When considering the arterial wall as viscoelastic, the above equation is modified by taking into account the viscous property of the wall,

$$\frac{c_o}{c} = (X - jY)(1 - jk_v \tan\phi) \qquad (4.5.44)$$

It has been shown that the viscous component is relatively small in large arteries, such as the aorta. The viscous loss represented by the magnitude of $\tan\phi$ is less than 10%.

Although in adequate, the Voigt model and the Maxwell model continues to be popular choices when taking into account of viscoelastic properties of the arterial wall. Womersley, as well as Morgan and Kiely (1954), and Jager *et al.* (1965) employed the Voigt model to describe the arterial wall properties. Jager *et al.* (1965) also assumed a thick-walled model, when the arterial wall thickness is a large fraction of the radius. A linearized Navier Stokes equation and dynamic deformation of the wall were also incorporated to arrive at a complex wave velocity:

$$c = \frac{Eh}{3\rho} \frac{2r+h}{(r+h)^2}(1 - F_{10}) \qquad (4.5.45)$$

In general, pressure and flow are obtained as periodic solutions with spatial and temporal dependences as:

$$p(z,t) = Me^{j\omega(t-z/c)} \qquad (4.5.46)$$

$$Q(z,t) = \frac{\pi r^2 M}{\rho c}(1 - F_{10})e^{j\omega(t-z/c)} \qquad (4.5.47)$$

Linear theories are based on certain assumptions as discussed in the previous section, they are mathematically tractable and allow solutions for pressure and flow to be expressed in closed forms.

4.5.3 *The Lumped Model of the Arterial System and the Windkessel Model*

The idea of a lumped model of the arterial circulation was first described by Hales in 1733. Albeit largely qualitative, he did emphasize the storage properties of large arteries and the dissipative nature of small peripheral resistance vessels. In his description, the blood ejected by the heart during systole into the arterial system distends the large arteries, primarily the aorta. During diastole, the elastic recoil of these same arteries propels blood to perfuse the smaller peripheral resistance vessels. This initiated the earlier conceptual understanding that the distensibility of large arteries is important in allowing the transformation of intermittent outflow of the heart to steady outflow throughout the peripheral vessels. In other words, the large overall "compliance" of the large arteries protects the stiff peripheral vessels of organ vascular beds from the large swing of blood pressure due to pulsations. This view is still held by many until this day. The significance of arterial pulsations remains a topic of debate.

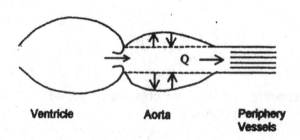

Ventricle   **Aorta**   **Periphery Vessels**

Fig. 4.5.2: Diagram representation of the left ventricle and the arterial circulation based on the idea of the Windkessel. The ventricle ejects into a compliant chamber representing the aorta, blood flow is stored in systole (solid line) and on elastic recoil in diastole (dotted line), the stiff peripheral vessels are perfused.

The Windkessel model is now credited to Frank (1899) whose original interest was in obtaining stroke volume from measured aortic pressure pulse contour. Methods to derive flow from pressure measurement or the so-termed pressure-derived flows (Li, 1983) have continued to attract considerable interest despite the advent of the electromagnetic blood flow and ultrasonic blood velocity measuring devices.

In the analysis of the Windkessel model, the amount of blood flow, Q_s, stored during each contraction is the difference between inflow, Q_i to the large arteries and the outflow, Q_o, to the small peripheral vessel (Fig. 4.5.2),

$$Q_s = Q_i - Q_o \qquad (4.5.48)$$

The amount of outflow is equivalent to the pressure drop from the arterial side (P) to the venous side (P_v) due to the peripheral resistance, R_s

$$Q_o = (P - P_v)/R_s \qquad (4.5.49)$$

At steady flow and assume that P_v is small, we obtain a familiar expression for estimating the peripheral resistance, and with the total inflow, $Q = Q_i$,

$$R_s = \overline{P} / \overline{Q} \qquad (4.5.50)$$

or mean arterial pressure to mean arterial flow.

The storage property can be described by the use of arterial compliance, which expresses the amount of change in blood volume (dV) due to a change in distending pressure (dP) in the arterial lumen. In this case, we have

$$C = dV/dP \qquad (4.5.51)$$

The amount of blood flow stored, or Q_s, due to arterial compliance, is related to the rate of change in pressure distending the artery,

$$Q_s = C \, dP/dt \qquad (4.5.52)$$

Substituting this equation and (4.5.49), we obtain from

$$Q_i = Q_s + Q_o \qquad (4.5.53)$$

an expression relating the arterial pressure to flow incorporating the two windkessel parameters, C and R_s:

$$Q(t) = C \, dP/dt + P/R_s \qquad (4.5.54)$$

In other words, the total arterial inflow is the sum of the flow stored in the aorta and the flow going into the periphery.

In diastole, when inflow is zero, as in the case when diastolic aortic flow equals zero after aortic valve closure, then

$$0 = C \, dP/dt + P/R_s \qquad (4.5.55)$$

or

$$dP/P = -dt/R_sC \qquad (4.5.56)$$

This equation states that the rate of diastolic aortic pressure drop is dependent on both the compliance of the arterial system and the total peripheral resistance. Both of which also determine the flow. Integration of both sides of equation (4.5.56) gives us

$$\ln P = t/R_sC \qquad (4.5.57)$$

or

$$P = P_0 \, e^{-t/R_sC} \qquad (4.5.58)$$

which is valid for the diastolic period, or $t = t_d$.

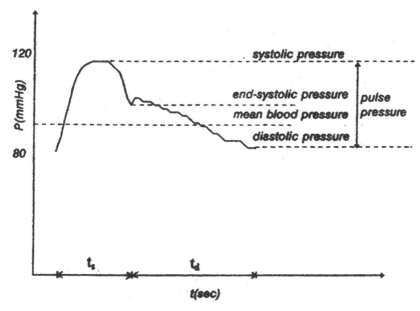

Fig. 4.5.3: Illustration of the measured aortic pressure pulse waveform. The systolic pressure, diastolic pressure, end-systolic pressure and mean blood pressure are also shown. The approximate exponential decay of diastolic pressure through the diastolic period (t_d) from the end of the systolic period (t_s) is seen.

This last equation is seen to be equivalent to

$$P_d = P_{es}\, e^{-td/\tau} \qquad (4.5.59)$$

or that the diastolic aortic pressure decay (Fig. 4.5.3) from end-systolic pressure ($P_{es)}$) to end-diastolic pressure (P_d) follows a mono-exponential manner with a time constant τ. The time constant of pressure decay, τ, is determined by the product of resistance and compliance, viz.

$$\tau = R_s C \qquad (4.5.60)$$

or in terms of measured aortic pressure,

$$\tau = \frac{t_d}{\ln \dfrac{P_{es}}{P_d}} \qquad (4.5.61)$$

and

$$C = \frac{t_d}{R_s \ln \frac{P_{es}}{P_d}} \tag{4.5.62}$$

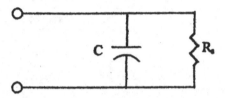

Fig. 4.5.4: The two-element resistance-capacitance electrical analog model of the Windkessel. Compliance is represented by a capacitor and the peripheral resistance by a resistor.

Analysis utilizing simple electric analog, has given the Windkessel a two-element representation. Arterial compliance is represented by a capacitor which has storage properties, in this case, electric charge. Peripheral resistance, with its viscous properties, is represented by a resistor which dissipates energy. This electrical analog of the Windkessel model of the arterial system is shown in Fig. 4.5.4.

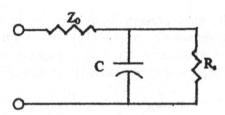

Fig. 4.5.5: An improved Windkessel with three-elements. Zo, represents the characteristic impedance aorta.

A modified Windkessel model (Fig. 4.5.5) that has three-elements was later proposed. This lumped model of the systemic arterial tree has been widely used. It consists of the total arterial compliance, the peripheral resistance and a characteristic impedance of the proximal aorta. Zo, as it is termed will be discussed in greater detail in a later section. Unlike the two-element model where input impedance approaches zero at high frequencies which is non-physiological, this model approximates better the input impedance of the vascular tree at higher frequencies with a constant value given by Zo.

Following the original work of representing the arterial system as transmission lines, the four-element model which is a section of the transmission line, has been proposed as a lumped model of the arterial system, as seen in Fig. 4.5.6. Here, the movement of blood mass or inertia effect is represented by an electrical inductor. That is, rate of changing flow contributes to alteration in pressure. Thus, the effect of blood flow acceleration, particularly in the aorta, becomes important. In the frequency domain, this four-element model approximates the input impedance better at higher frequencies, particularly the oscillatory parts. It should be noted here this 4-element is reduced to the 3-element, given that $Zo=(L/R)^{1/2}$.

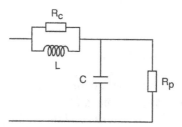

Fig. 4.5.6: A four-element lumped model of the arterial system. The inertial effect is represented by an inductor which can be placed in series or in parallel, to the resistance.

For all practical purposes in terms of actual fluid flow, a hydraulic equivalent is more useful. Figure 4.5.7 illustrates such a model. Here the left ventricle is simulated with an elastic pump which is connected to a solenoid whose timing can be adjusted to control the inflow to the arterial system.

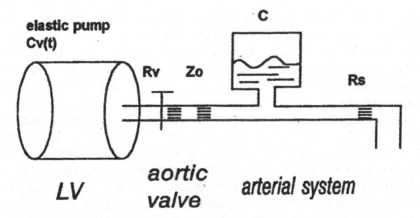

Fig. 4.5.7: The hydraulic equivalent of the three-element Windkessel, popularly used to represent the arterial load to the heart. A bottle allowing volume displacement subjecting to pressure variations represents the arterial compliance. The peripheral resistance is represented by a needle valve whose partial opening and closing allows resistance to flow to be varied. The finite tube geometry and property represents the characteristic impedance of the aorta.

4.5.4 *Nonlinear Aspects and Pressure-Dependent Arterial Compliance*

Although the Navier-Stokes equation in its complete form has recently been solved in closed form (Melbin and Noordergraaf, 1983), there are other kinds of nonlinearities. Thus, depending on the particular problem or application at hand, assumptions included in order to eliminate some or all of the nonlinearities may still be valid to provide a satisfactory solution. This is particularly true with regard to the use of Fourier analysis in studying pressure and flow waveforms and the derived input impedance analysis.

The general definition of arterial compliance is the ratio of an incremental change in volume due to an incremental change in distending pressure, i.e.

$$C = dV/dP \qquad (4.5.63)$$

This is defined by the inverse of the slope of the pressure-volume (P-V) curve, with pressure plotted on the ordinate and volume on the abscissa (Fig. 4.5.8). Thus, compliance is the inverse of stiffness.

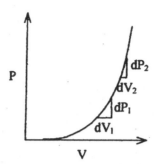

Fig. 4.5.8: Arterial pressure-volume diagram, defining compliance as the slope of the relation (C=dV/dP). It is clear that the slope changes with increasing pressure (dV_1/dP_1 vs. dV_2/dP_1) and at higher pressures the volume change is smaller.

The pressure-volume curves of arteries have been found to be curvilinear. The slope changes along the P-V curve steeper at higher pressures, signifying increased arterial stiffness or decreased compliance and distensibility. In other words, arteries stiffen when pressurized. This physiological phenomenon has been observed in many experiments. This increased stiffness has been suggested to be related to the structure of the arterial wall. This implies that the compliance-pressure relation is not a constant one. The declining arterial compliance with increasing pressure has been observed in the central aorta and in individual arteries. The inverse exponential relation between compliance and pressure for the arterial system is shown in Fig. 4.5.9.

A nonlinear model of the arterial system incorporating a pressure-dependent compliance element *(C(P))* is shown in Fig. 4.5.10 (Li *et al.*, 1990). The model consists of the characteristic impedance of the proximal aorta (Z_o), the peripheral resistance (R_s), and *C(P)*. The compliance is exponentially related to pressure and is expressed as

$$C(P) = a \cdot e^{b(P(t))} \qquad (4.5.64)$$

where a and b are constants. The exponent b is normally negative. Thus, an inverse relationship is established between arterial compliance and blood pressure; with increasing blood pressure arterial compliance decreases.

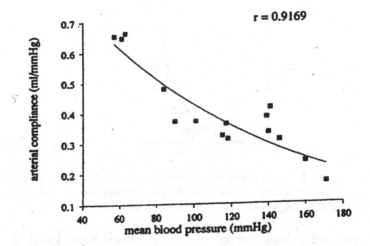

Fig. 4.5.9: Compliance plotted against mean arterial blood pressure reflecting the pressure-volume relation. The relationship is nonlinear, implying that at higher distending pressures the intraluminal volume change is smaller, resulting in a lower compliance. The decrease in arterial compliance with increasing blood pressure follows a negative exponential function.

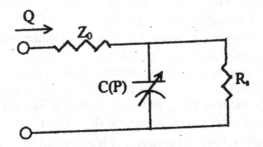

Fig. 4.5.10: Nonlinear arterial system model according to Li *et al.* (1990), incorporating a pressure-dependent compliance. Z_0 is characteristic impedance of the ascending aorta, R_s is total peripheral resistance, C(P) is the pressure-dependent compliance, represented by a variable capacitor. Q is aortic flow.

Figure 4.5.10 shows that the flow through the compliance branch of the nonlinear model is given by

$$Q_c(t) = Q(t) - P(t)/R_s \qquad (4.5.65)$$

where P(t) and Q(t) are the pressure and flow through the compliance branch, respectively. This flow can also be expressed as

$$Q_c(t) = C(P) \cdot dP(t)/dt \qquad (4.5.66)$$

Equate these two equations, resulting in

$$dP/dt = (Q(t) - P(t)/R_s)/C(P) \qquad (4.5.67)$$

This equation defines the dynamic relationship between pressure and flow for a nonlinear compliance element. Numerical methods can be employed to solve this equation.

Using difference representations, we have

$$\Delta t = t_{i+1} - t_i = dt \qquad (4.5.68)$$

where Δt is the sampling interval, taken as 10 msec. The nonlinear model is then reduced to the following expression:

$$P(t_{i+1}) = P(t_i) + \Delta t \cdot (Q(t_i) - P(t_i)/R_s)/C(P) \qquad (4.5.69)$$

With the measured aortic flow as the input, a numerical procedure can be programmed to solve P(t$_j$), C(P) and the aortic pressure

$$P_a(t_i) = Q(t_i) \cdot Z_o + P(t_i) \qquad (4.5.70)$$

This nonlinear model predicted aortic pressure accurately, as shown in Fig. 4.5.11. The linear three-element model predicted the measured aortic pressure with less accuracy, although the gross features are evident. The model-based arterial compliance plotted as a function of pressure for a complete cardiac cycle with a normal blood pressure level is shown in Fig. 4.5.12. It is clear from this figure that compliance is relatively independent of both pressure and flow in the early systole and maintains a value close to its maximum during this period. This facilitates early rapid ventricular ejection. During mid-systole, arterial compliance declines, corresponding to increased aortic pressure and reduced ejection after peak ventricular outflow. In the late systolic phase, arterial compliance declines rapidly with a concurrent rapid decline of aortic flow, despite a falling aortic pressure. The compliance value is much higher at early systole than at late systole. Arterial system compliance reaches its minimum at the end of the ejection. For the diastolic period, when aortic flow is zero, compliance follows an exponential relation as given by equation (4.5.64). Its value increases throughout the diastole towards maximum, readying for the following ventricular ejection. The pressure-dependent compliance behaviors in the time and frequency domains were analyzed in considerable by Matonick and Li (2001).

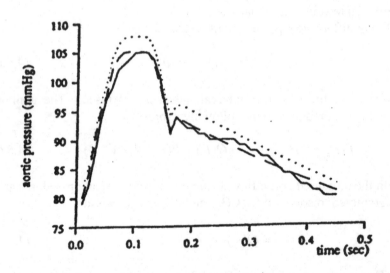

Fig. 4.5.11: The nonlinear and linear model predicted aortic pressure waveforms, compared to the measured aortic pressure. Dotted line: linear Windkessel model; dashed line: nonlinear pressure-dependent compliance model.

Recent work in our group based on the Wiener system model (Patel *et al.*, 2016) affords good prediction of the central aortic pressure waveform from the measurements of two peripheral arterial pressures.

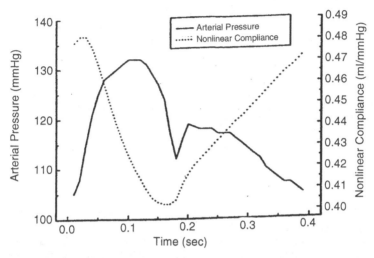

Fig. 4.5.12: Nonlinear pressure-dependent characteristics of arterial compliance as a function of time plotted for a complete cardiac cycle. Arterial compliance increases initially at the beginning of ejection and declines with increasing pressure. It reaches a minimum at about end-systole and increases steadily thence towards the end of diastole.

Arterial compliance and blood pressure bears a close relation. As such the beat-to-beat pressure-compliance loop actually represents a logical new approach to describing blood vessel properties. It allows visualization of vessel lumen geometry changes in relation to mechanical property alteration throughout the cardiac cycle (Li, 1998). This can be well illustrated when the compliance-pressure loops for control, methoxamine induced hypertension and vasodilation induced profound vasodilation are plotted on a single graph as illustrated in Fig. 4.5.13. Here the compliance change over the entire range of pressure (50-200 mmHg) is clearly seen, i.e. compliance decreases with increasing pressure. More importantly, the range of compliance variation within a cardiac cycle is significantly compressed in hypertension despite large distending pressure (150-200 mmHg), indicating increased vascular stiffness. In contrast, vasodilation with nitroprusside is associated with a large compliance-pressure loop area, accompanied by significantly increased compliance. Increased lumen area is also expected.

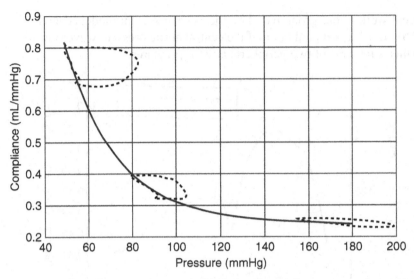

Fig. 4.5.13: Compliance vs pressure (solid line) and compliance-pressure loops (dotted lines) plotted for the control (middle), methoxamine induced hypertension (right) and nitroprusside induced vasodilation (left) cases. Notice the overall compliance decreases with increasing pressure and that the loop area is compressed in hypertension and enlarged with vasodilator.

In describing fluid motions with a linearized Navier-Stokes equation, nonlinear terms are assumed to be small and are consequently neglected. Ling *et al.* (1973) Computed flows from an accurately measured pressure gradient (with a claimed resolution of 0.001 mmHg). They found that linear theory overestimated the steady flow term by several folds, while the pulsatile flow waveforms conformed rather well with electromagnetically measured flow. Li *et al.* (1981) measured the propagation constant in arteries and found that the measured attenuation coefficients and phase velocities differed greatly from those predicted by linear theories. To explain the observed discrepancies, they evaluated and compared the nonlinear and linear theories for the femoral artery. For the nonlinear theory, the complete solution of the Navier-Stokes equation, the geometric taper, and pressure-dependent wall compliance were incorporated. Although varied nonlinearities have been incorporated in some nonlinear theories, in general vascular branching has not been included. Its effect is significant in pulse transmission. This aspect will be discussed in the following chapter.

Chapter 5

Vascular Branching

5.1 Branching Geometry

5.1.1 *Complexity of Vascular Branching*

The branching geometry of the vascular network has intrigued investigators for centuries. Its complexity and precise arrangement of the large vessels and their connectivity to the vast number of small microcirculatory vessels have amazed scientists and clinicians alike. The intermingling of geometric architecture and the mechanical properties of the vascular structure at branching points is of particular interest in this Chapter.

To perfuse organ vascular beds and meet specific tissue metabolic demands, the vascular system displays its utmost efficient transport network structure through branching of blood vessels. This allows prompt spatial and temporal distribution of oxygen and nutrients and removal of waste products. One would marvel the vascular system of the human heart, for instance, with its own well-meshed branching circulation, the coronary circulation, to supply its own blood according to its own energetic demand and mechanical performance. The lungs, with its branching pulmonary vascular tree give another example of achieving the functional requirement of ventilation-perfusion, on demand. The complex branching topology of the cerebral circulation to supply oxygen and blood flow to neuronal networks and the extensive network of vessels in the renal circulation, are just some of the examples one can marvel the branching topology and structure of the vascular system.

Branching of blood vessels can be viewed as a simple consequence of the necessity in providing an efficient vascular network for distribution of fluid flow, in this case, blood flow. In terms of angiogenesis, however, vascular endothelial growth factor-A or VEGF-A, has been recognized to play a role at the cellular level in the formation of vascular network. Hemodynamic forces naturally follow. But the simplest form of branching is through bifurcation. A vascular structure of this form in which the mother or source vessel is bifurcating into two daughter or branching vessels, undergoes further bifurcation for generations. This is known as the "open tree" structure. In such simplistic and idealistic representation, each of the branching vessels is of the same lumen diameter and the same vessel length. In addition, the angle of bifurcation maintains the same. Thus, this uniform bifurcating structure represents a basic fractal-like tree network model of the vascular system. Theoretical studies based on bifurcation geometry have been numerous. The outcome from their predictions has been mixed. Good correlations have been found for the extent of bifurcation vessel lengths and diameters, much less for bifurcation angles, optimally at about 75° for an equi-bifurcation on theoretical grounds (Iberall, 1967) and experimental measurements (Li, 1984). A different finding of how flow is optimized through bifurcation angles in the coronary vasculature was provided by Huo *et al.* (2012).

Vascular networks and branching geometry however are far more complex in the cardiovascular system. And from the imaging standpoint of view, most vascular branches do not lie on the same plan of view. This makes 3-D reconstruction of vascular topology from 2-D images somewhat challenging. Although bifurcation is the most common form of vascular branching, trifurcation and multi-branching junctions also occur in the mammalian vascular systems. In addition, the uniformity in geometry is often not observed. That is, branching vessel diameters and lengths, as well as branching angles can vary considerably. Nevertheless, bifurcation predominates in the vascular branching structure.

Examples of the vascular branching structure that do not obey the straight bifurcation scheme is readily visible by looking at the aorta and its branches. The aortic arch is curved and has many branches, none of which maintains the same vessel diameter and length in these branching arteries, such as the brachiocephalic and the subclavian. However, the two common carotid arteries represent a long, uniform, bifurcating structure. Taking the direction along the length of the thoracic aorta through abdominal aorta, we observe many branches that come off the aorta at almost right angles, far from those at the aortic arch or the aorto-iliac junction. Segmental arteries that help to perfuse the spinal cord, come off mostly at right angles from the descending aorta. The aorta however, provides another kind of branching structure for efficient transport. For instance, the aorta itself, though tapered, maintains a larger trunk diameter in comparison to its branching arteries and its dominating length ensures fast delivery of blood to its branches. This represents another scheme of branching structure.

5.1.2 Nonuniform Branching and 3-D Branching Structures

The above considerations of branching structure are not limited to two-dimensional (2-D) vascular networks. In the 2-D structure, all blood vessels lie in the same plane. A three-dimensional (3-D) structure allows greater flexibility and expansion. Adding on the nonuniform scheme, the vascular tree has even greater flexibility in defining its structure.

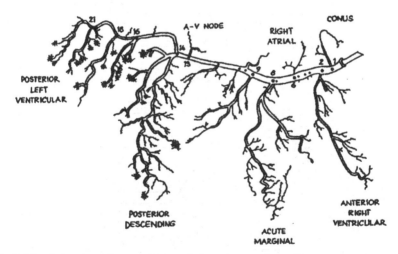

Fig. 5.1.1: A drawing of some of the main branches coming off from the right coronary artery as it circles the heart. Numbers refer to vascular junctions along the artery. From Zamir (2000).

Morphological structures of the branching vascular systems have been reported by numerous investigators. One such an example is shown in Fig. 5.1.1, given by Zamir (2000). The main vessel branches from the right coronary artery are shown, together with the numbers that identify branching junctions as they arise sequentially along the coronary artery. These numbers are related to the levels of the arterial tree as illustrated schematically in Fig. 5.1.2. This is used for mapping the branches arising at these junctions. This scheme clearly shows the tree structure that is nonuniform and incomplete in terms of the order of branching to terminations 5.1.3). Both the number of junctions and the level or the tree, are clearly defined.

There are other differing branching structures found in the special circulations. For instances, the morphometry in the pig coronary venous system by Kassab *et al.* (1993) and the network anatomy of arteries feeding the spinotrapezius muscle in both normal and hypertensive rats by Schmid-Shonbein *et al.* (1986) differ considerably.

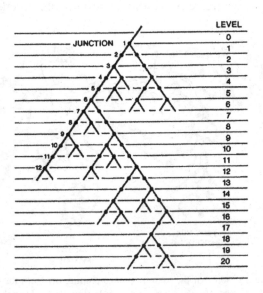

Fig. 5.1.2: Schematic drawing of the tree structure corresponding to the previous figure showing the number of junctions and levels.

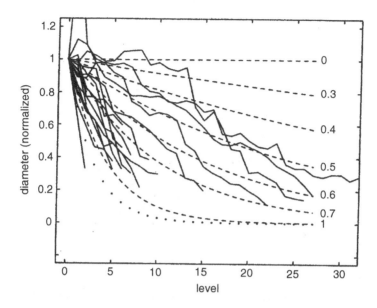

Fig. 5.1.3: Changes in normalized diameter along the right coronary artery and some of its main branches. The bifurcation index is shown on the right. Dotted line: square-law; dashed lines: cube-law. From Zamir (2000).

5.1.3 *Space-Filling Properties and Modeling*

It is known that the greater the body surface area, the greater the need for an expansion of vascular networks to perfuse the tissues. Many cardiac indices have therefore, been normalized to body surface area. With a given organ vascular bed, space-filling is then a property, whether in terms of area-expansion or volume-filling.

One approach takes into consideration of the space-filling problem is the structured tree model shown in Fig. 5.1.4. Here small arteries and arterioles exercise minimization principles to perfuse tissues with blood. Olufsen (2000) modeled branching small arteries and large arterioles with the termination reached when the arterioles reach a prescribed minimal radius. The determinants of the structured tree model are the scaling parameters α (<1) and β (<1), the order of the tree and the geometric and elastic properties of the vessels. Results show the pressure and flow waveforms manifested in large arteries have similar forms to the measured data.

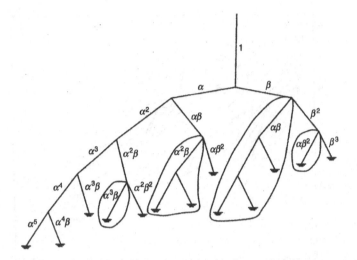

Fig. 5.1.4: A structured tree model in which at each bifurcation the radii of the daughter vessels are scaled linearly by factors α and β, respectively. From Olufsen (2000).

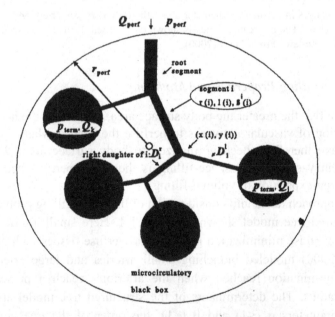

Fig. 5.1.5: A schematic drawing of the constrained constructive optimization, showing perfusion through the root segment and blood delivery by terminal segments at four randomly chosen locations within a given perfusion area. From Schreiner *et al.* (2000).

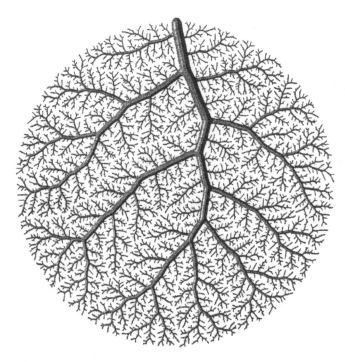

Fig. 5.1.6: Constrained constructive optimization obtained vascular tree network with 4,000 terminal segments generated in a 2-D perfusion area. Minimum intravascular volume is optimized at bifurcation exponent of k=3. No minimum symmetry is assumed. From Schreiner *et al.* (2000).

Another approach to examine the branching structure of blood vessels is through the constrained constructive optimization. This technique has been shown to be able to generate realistic models of arterial trees involving thousands of vascular segments. An example is given by Schreiner *et al.* (2000), shown in Fig. 5.1.5. Here, a drawing of the constrained constructive optimization scheme is displayed, showing perfusion through the root segment and blood delivery by terminal segments at four randomly chosen locations within a given perfusion area. Further, the bifurcation scheme is utilized where the radii of the mother (m) and daughter (d_1, d_2) vessel segments at each bifurcation follows:

$$r_m{}^k = r_{d1}{}^k + r_{d2}{}^k \qquad (5.1.1)$$

It has been shown that $2 \le k \le 3$ are physiologically relevant. Fig. 5.1.6 illustrates one such result after structural optimization is applied, assuming k=3.

5.2 Fluid Mechanics of Vascular Branching

5.2.1 Branching Geometry and Fluid Dynamic Considerations

There are numerous branching junctions in the vascular system. Bifurcations are the most common. Some of these are, for instances, aorta to left and right iliac arteries or aorto-iliac bifurcation, common carotid to internal and external carotid arteries or carotid artery bifurcation, the femoral artery bifurcation, the celiac artery bifurcation, mesenteric bifurcation and coronary artery bifurcations.

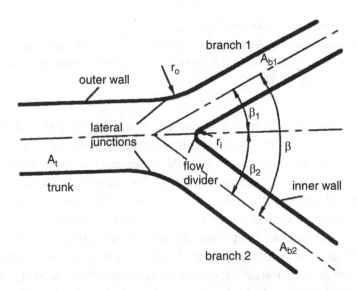

Fig. 5.2.1: Branching morphology with Y-shaped bifurcating tubes. The source or trunk vessel gives rise into two branches. A = cross sectional area, β = angle of branching or bifurcation angle, r = radius of curvature.

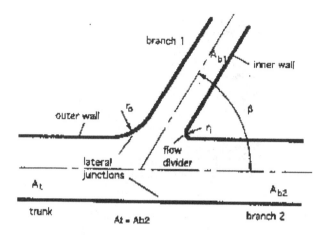

Fig. 5.2.2: Main vessel with a side branch or T-shaped bifurcation. One of the branching vessel has the same cross sectional area as the source vessel.

Bio-fluid dynamics for various arterial bifurcations have been intensively investigated. In the studies of bifurcations, two general shapes, such as T-shaped and Y-shaped branching morphology have been used (Lou and Yang, 1992). The aortic, carotid, iliac and coronary bifurcations are considered Y-shaped, while renal femoral, celiac and mesenteric branching are considered T-shaped in fluid mechanical studies. These are illustrated in Figs. 5.2.1 and 5.2.2.

The importance of area ratios is dealt in the next section. Area ratios and curvatures of flow divider and lateral junctions are major geometric parameters considered in the formulation of many fluid mechanical studies. Li (1986) has found that alteration of pressure and flow through vascular junctions is more significantly affected by geometry than by elastic factors.

The effect of flow divider curvature was studied in a numerical simulation model by Friedman and Ehrlich (1984). Two-dimensional steady flow calculation in computational regions obtained from radiographs of human aortic bifurcations have been shown to correlate well with unsteady measurements of wall shear in flow-through casts of the same vessels. Their results suggest that wall slope, hence curvature is an important factor affecting shear that contributes to atherogenesis. This approach is shown in Figs. 5.2.3 and 5.2.4.

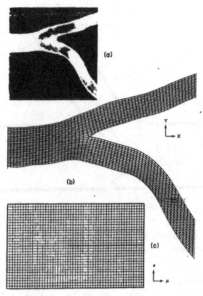

Fig. 5.2.3: Transformation of branch geometry to a rectangular mesh: (a) frontal-plane radiograph of the bifurcations, (b) the untransformed grid in the X-Y plane obtained from the radiograph, (c) the transformed grid in the u-v plane where the inner wall have been mapped onto the horizontal slit. From Friedman and Ehrlich (1984).

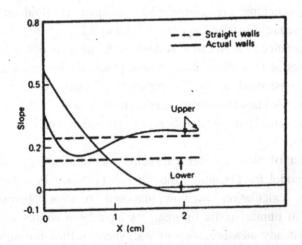

Fig. 5.2.4: Slope profile along the actual and straight inner walls. Since the end points of the straight walls are the same as those of the corresponding actual walls, the slopes of the straightened walls are equal to the mean slopes of the actual walls. From Friedman and Ehrlich (1984).

Many of fluid mechanical simulations and experiments in branching tubes have taken the assumption of rigid tubes. We have seen in earlier chapters that blood vessel compliance is of utmost importance in shaping the pressure and flow waveforms.

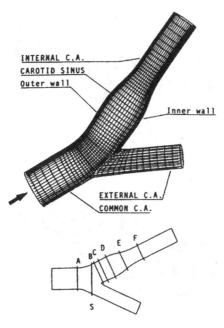

Fig. 5.2.5: Carotid bifurcation model. A, B, C, D, E, F, S indicate flow cross-section levels where numerical results are displayed. From Perktold and Rappitsch (1995).

One such study that addresses the importance of compliance is that of Perktold and Rappitsch (1995) who performed computer simulation of local blood flow and vessel mechanics in a compliant carotid artery bifurcation model. The flow analysis uses the time-dependent, three-dimensional, incompressible Navier-Stokes equations for non-Newtonian inelastic fluids. The wall displacement and stress analysis applies geometrically nonlinear shell theory where incrementally linear elastic wall property is assumed. Their comparison of rigid and compliant vessel models showed that wall shear stress magnitude decreased by 25% in the

compliant model.   In general, flow separation results in locally low
oscillating wall shear stress. These are illustrated in Figs. 5.2.5, 5.2.6 and
5.2.7. Carotid bifurcation has also been studied, for instances, by laser
Doppler anemometer measurements of pulsatile flow in a model (Ku and
Giddens, 1987) and in a three-dimensional analysis (Gilsen *et al.*, 1999).

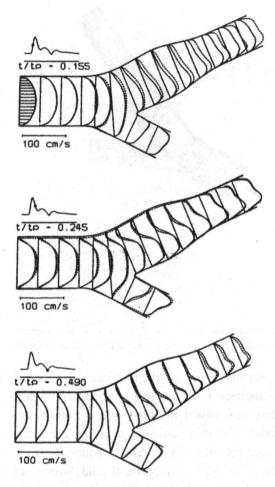

Fig. 5.2.6: Axial flow velocity profiles at the symmetry plane during systolic contraction
phase (top), systolic deceleration phase (middle) and the pulse phase of minimum flow
rate (bottom). Solid line: compliant model; dashed line: rigid model. From Perktold and
Rappitsch (1995).

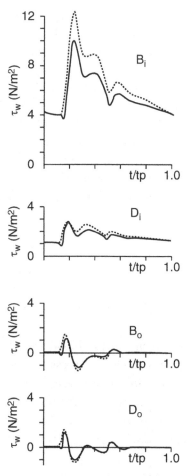

Fig. 5.2.7: Wall shear stress during the pulse cycle at the inner wall (internal divider wall) Bi, Di and at the outer internal wall Bo, Do. Solid line: compliant model; dashed line: rigid model. From Perktold and Rappitsch (1995).

5.2.2 *Fluid Mechanics Associated with Atherosclerosis and Stenosis*

The susceptibility of vascular branches to atherosclerosis is believed due in part to the unusual fluid dynamic environments that the vessel wall experiences in the regions. Fluid mechanical studies have shown that atherosclerosis may occur at branching points where the geometry is complex, a large Reynolds number and a lower than average wall shear stress. In general, the complex flow pattern is associated with a spatially nonuniform shear stress and wall curvature. The rate of change of shear stress and shear rate have been shown to be important, as well as local turbulence and unsteady flow. In addition local disturbed flow patterns, recirculation zones, long particle residence times have been suggested to play significant roles in the onset and development of atherosclerosis.

Numerous modeling and experimental studies have been proposed to investigate the fluid mechanical factors contributing to atherosclerosis. Caro *et al.* (1971) were earlier investigators to identify sites of atherogenesis as regions of reduced wall shear stress (Caro, 2009) and suggested that the transport of lipoprotein within the arterial wall and across the endothelium is a major factor in atherosclerosis. These common atherosclerotic sites have been illustrated by DeBakey *et al.* (1985). Numerical simulation to predict some of these branching sites has been carried in a two-dimensional simulation (Lei *et al.*, 1995). Friedman (1989) used a model to explain the thickening of arterial intima under shear. Thurbrikar and Robicsec (1995) suggested the importance of pressure-induced arterial wall stress as an important factor in atherosclerosis.

Stenosis, or the narrowing of the blood vessel, is associated with a serious hemodynamic consequence of pressure loss that develops across the stenosis. The pressure loss is primarily dependent on the flow rate and the geometry of the stenosis, since the fluid properties of density and apparent viscosity are relatively constant. The fluid mechanics aspect of stenosis has been well studied, owing to its importance in the coronary arteries (e.g. Mates *et al.*, 1978).

Arteries with severe stenoses caused by atherosclerotic plague growth may collapse under physiological conditions (Aorki and Ku, 1993). Artery collapse is a process where an artery buckles under certain pressure and stress conditions. The compression resulting from this collapse may lead to accelerated fatigue and rupture of the fibrous cap, which contains the plague. The plague rupture can lead directly to heart attack and stroke if occurring in coronary and cerebral vessels, respectively. It is known that local stenosis formed by an atherosclerotic lesion may cause mechanical conditions favorable for artery collapse. Plague fatigue and distal embolization are also important considerations.

Blood flow must accelerate to high velocities in the narrowed stenosis. The high velocities in turn create a low or negative transmural pressure, which can result in collapse of the artery. Alternatively, the high velocities at the stenosis also generate high shear stresses, which may be related to plague cap rupture and platelet activation (Tang *et al.*, 1999). It has been shown that the pulsatile blood flow characteristics, as we discussed in earlier chapters, cannot be neglected, particularly in the evolution of vortex structures downstream from the stenosis. It is essential to determine the wall shear stress temporal evolution downstream from a stenosis.

The close relation of atherosclerosis and stenosis and their morphological resemblance have indeed generated much interest in analyzing common fluid mechanical factors and consequences. In many instances, particularly in modeling studies, these two pathological conditions cannot be separated. Their importance in the manifestation of eventual diseases of the vascular system, however, is well recognized. Tarbell *et al.* (2014) provided a comprehensive review of the relationships of fluid mechanics to arterial diseases, as well as the role of gene expression.

5.3 Pulse Transmission Characteristics at Vascular Branching

5.3.1 *Impedance Matching and Wave Reflections*

One consequence of vascular branching is the pronounced changes in pressure and flow waveforms. To this end, analysis of pulse transmission characteristics at vascular branching has been limited. Pulse transmission at branching junction, unlike that along a single continuous vessel, depends on the mechanical and geometric properties of the source or mother vessel as well as on the branching or daughter vessels. Impedance is an effective means to embrace all these properties. If the combined impedances of the daughter vessel match that of the mother vessel, then, the transmission will simply be ideal and there will be no wave reflections, nor energetic losses at the branching junction.

The relations for the pressure and flow pulse waveforms expressed as magnitude and phase are, as defined previously, for the nth harmonic:

$$P_n = |P_n| e^{j(\omega t + \phi_n)} \qquad (5.3.1)$$

$$Q_n = |Q_n| e^{j(\omega t + \varphi_n)} \qquad (5.3.2)$$

The vascular impedance obtained for the nth harmonic is therefore,

$$Z_n = |Z_n| e^{j\theta_n} \qquad (5.3.3)$$

where the magnitude of impedance is simply the ratio of the pressure amplitude to the flow amplitude, and for the nth harmonic:

$$|Z_n| = \frac{|P_n|}{|Q_n|} \qquad (5.3.4)$$

with the phase lag

$$\theta_n = \phi_n - \varphi_n \qquad (5.3.5)$$

Characteristic impedance that reflect the vessel properties alone, irrespective of wave reflections can then be approximated from the high frequency average of the impedance modulus. Characteristic impedance, like input impedance, is complex, although its dependence on frequency is only weakly so in large vessels.

In order to isolate the contributions of vascular branching to overall pulse transmission characteristics, it is necessary to define local characteristic impedances that reflect the mechanical and geometric properties of the vessels at vascular junction.

A local reflection coefficient can be defined for vascular branching only:

$$\Gamma_l = \frac{Z_{od} - Z_{om}}{Z_{od} + Z_{om}} \qquad (5.3.6)$$

Where Z_{od} represents the resultant parallel combination of the characteristic impedance of branching daughter vessels, and Z_{om} is the mother vessel's characteristic impedance. For instance, for a bifurcation with daughter branch characteristic impedances of Z_{o1} and Z_{o2}, we have:

$$\frac{1}{Z_{od}} = \frac{1}{Z_{o1}} + \frac{1}{Z_{o2}}$$ (5.3.7)

For an equi-bifurcation (Fig. 5.3.1), one obtains:

$$\frac{1}{Z_{od}} = \frac{1}{Z_{o1}} + \frac{1}{Z_{o2}} = \frac{2}{Z_{o1}}$$ (5.3.8)

In terms of the mother or source vessel characteristic impedance, Z_{om}, and individual daughter or branch vessel characteristic impedance, Z_{o1}, we obtain for the local wave reflection due to equi-vascular branching only:

$$\Gamma_l = \frac{Z_{o1} - 2Z_{om}}{Z_{o1} + 2Z_{om}}$$ (5.3.9)

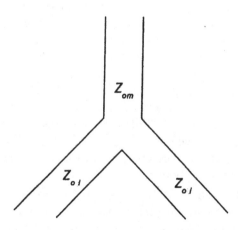

Fig. 5.3.1: Schematic representation of a branching vascular junction, An equi-bifurcation is illustrated with characteristic impedance of the mother (Z_{om}) and daughter (Z_{o1}) vessels respectively.

An alternative method that assumes frequency independence of characteristic impedance, is derived from the water-hammer formula (Li, 1985). In this formulation, the pressure and flow are expressed as:

$$P = \rho \cdot v \cdot c \tag{5.3.10}$$

$$Q = v \cdot \pi r^2 \tag{5.3.11}$$

The characteristic impedance is defined simply by the ratio of pressure to flow, i.e.

$$Z_o = \frac{\rho c}{\pi r^2} \tag{5.3.12}$$

This gives the characteristic impedance of a uniform cylindrical vessel that is independent of wave reflections. Of course, the blood flow is assumed to be Newtonian and that the viscosity of blood and the vessels wall are neglected in this formulation.

5.3.2 *Area Ratio Concept*

From a simple geometric perspective, the cross-sectional area of the adjoining vessels should provide some quantitative estimates of the mismatching characteristics of pulse transmission characteristics. Thus, the branching vessel lumen areas come into play. This concept of area ratio has been examined by several investigators. For instance, Karreman (1952) used area ratio in his mathematical formulation of wave reflection at an arterial junction. By assuming both the wall and fluid are nonviscous, and wall thickness remains the same for an infinitely long tube, he arrived at a value of area ratio (the ratio of the sum of the areas of daughter vessels to that of the mother vessel) for a reflectionless bifurcation of about 1.15.

With a modification by considering tethered elastic tubes containing viscous fluid, Womersley (1958) later arrived at a similar result with a correcting factor q, for a bifurcation, assuming the daughter vessels have identical characteristics (r_d, c_d):

$$A_b = 2 \cdot \left(\frac{r_d}{r_m}\right)^2 \left(\frac{c_m}{c_d}\right) \cdot q \qquad (5.3.13)$$

The local reflection coefficient due to the equi-bifurcation is then given by:

$$\Gamma_l = \frac{1 - A_b}{1 + A_b} \qquad (5.3.14)$$

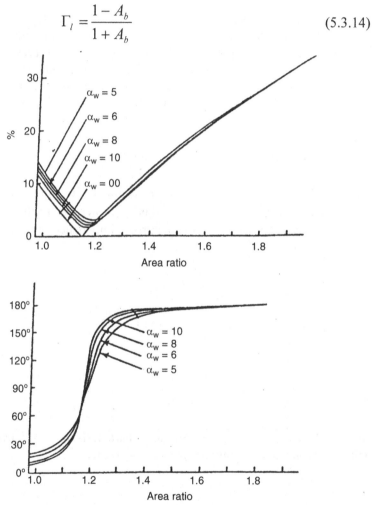

Fig. 5.3.2: Reflections at vascular branching. Magnitude and phase of local reflection coefficients computed for an equi-bifurcation are plotted against area ratios. From Womersley (1958).

Exact matching is not possible. Perfect matching is only obtained when the Womersley's number,

$$\alpha_\omega = r\sqrt{\frac{\omega\rho}{\eta}} \qquad (5.3.15)$$

approaches infinity, or $\alpha_\omega \to \infty$, though the minimum reflection is only a few percent. This is shown in Fig. 5.3.2. The area ratios for the aortic junctions are usually between 1.15 and 1.25, which represent a very small amount of reflections (Li *et al.*, 1984). These same small amount of local reflections were found on the analog model of the systemic arterial tree by Westerhof *et al.* (1969). In terms of fluid dynamics, optimal energy transfer is achieved when the area ratio is close to one, as found here.

The relationship of local reflection coefficient, area ratio and junction vessel characteristic impedances can be easily appreciated from the following analysis. We first relate the characteristic impedance of the blood vessel to its geometric and elastic properties. From the water-hammer formula above for the characteristic impedance, we have

$$Z_o = \frac{\rho c}{\pi r^2} \qquad (5.3.16)$$

Knowing the Moens-Korteweg relation (1.1.1), $A = \pi r^2$ and substituting for pulse wave velocity, c, we have:

$$Z_o = \frac{1}{A}\sqrt{\frac{Eh\rho}{2r}} \qquad (5.3.17)$$

Now with a bifurcation, the resultant characteristic impedance of the daughter vessel branch impedances, Z_1 and Z_2, is:

$$\frac{1}{Z_d} = \frac{1}{Z_1} + \frac{1}{Z_2} \qquad (5.3.18)$$

For an equi-bifurcation, or $Z_2 = Z_1$, we have

$$\frac{1}{Z_d} = \frac{2}{Z_1} \qquad (5.3.19)$$

or for n equal daughter branches:

$$\frac{1}{Z_d} = \frac{n}{Z_1} \qquad (5.3.20)$$

The fraction of the pressure pulse that is reflected at the junction due to unmatched branching vessel characteristic impedances is

$$\Gamma_l = \frac{Z_d - Z_m}{Z_d + Z_m} = \frac{1 - Z_m / Z_d}{1 + Z_m / Z_d} \qquad (5.3.21)$$

where Z_m and Z_d are the characteristic impedances of the mother and daughter vessels, respectively.

This latter leads to a junction reflection of

$$\Gamma_l = \frac{1 - n Z_m / Z_1}{1 + n Z_m / Z_1} \qquad (5.3.22)$$

If we let

$$Z_m = \frac{\rho c_m}{A_m} \text{ and } Z_1 = \frac{\rho c_1}{A_1} \qquad (5.3.23)$$

then, for n equal branches, we obtain

$$\frac{Z_m}{Z_d} = n \cdot \frac{A_1}{A_m} \cdot \frac{c_m}{c_1} \qquad (5.3.24)$$

where

$$A_r = n \cdot \frac{A_1}{A_m} \qquad (5.3.25)$$

is the area ratio (A_r) and c_m/c_1 is the velocity ratio, related to the ratio of elastic properties of the branching vessels:

$$\frac{c_m}{c_1} = \sqrt{\frac{E_m}{E_1}} \qquad (5.3.26)$$

This assumes that the wall thickness-to-radius ratio or h/r is relatively constant for the branching vessels.

Since

$$A_r = n \cdot \left(\frac{r_1}{r_m}\right)^2 \qquad (5.3.27)$$

it is clear that alterations in branching vessel lumen radii could exert a more significant effect on wave reflections at vascular branching junction, Γ_l, than changes in their respective elastic moduli.

For constant elasticity for all vessels involved at vascular branching, i.e. $c_m/c_1 = 1$, the wave reflections due to vascular branching becomes dependent only on area ratio, i.e.

$$\Gamma_l = \frac{1 - A_r}{1 + A_r} \qquad (5.3.28)$$

5.3.3 *Minimum Local Reflections at Vascular Branching Junctions*

By examination of the characteristic impedances of mother and daughter vessels, that pulse wave reflection due to vascular branching is minimal (Li, 1984). Since reflection is energetically wasteful, this means little energy is lost due to pulse transmission through vascular branching junctions. This has been attributed to close to optimal area ratios and branching angles. Also geometric effect rather than elastic effect dominants pulse propagation through vascular branching junctions (Li, 1986).

The area ratio concept has received continued attention. Experimental results showed that minimum reflection is obtained when area ratio equals 1.23 for an equi-bifurcation. This correlates closely to that given by Womersley's theory (minimum reflection when area ratio equals 1.26). In small muscular vessels, viscous damping is appreciably more important than in large vessels. In these vessels, the point of minimum reflection (in the reflection vs. area ratio plot) is shifted to a larger area ratio, accompanied by a larger phase change.

The importance of topological geometry and elastic properties at vascular branching junctions can be easily appreciated from the measurement of local reflection coefficients involving characteristic impedances of junction vessels. By using measured and calculated vascular parameters (Table 5.3.1) obtained from measurements in dog aorto-iliac junction (a trifurcation with the abdominal aorta branching into its continuation branch and left and right iliac arteries), the local reflection was found to be just 0.07 (Li, 1984, 1986).

Table 5.3.1: Measured and Calculated Vascular Parameters.

	A cm^2	c cm/s	Z_0 dyn.s.cm^{-5}	E 10^6dyn/cm^2
Abdominal aorta	0.415	660	1686	5.54
Continuation branch	0.205	710	3671	6.41
Iliac artery	0.115	765	7051	7.44

Figure 5.3.3 shows that the local reflection coefficient is significantly increased when the vessel lumen radius is progressively decreased downstream from the junction (daughter vessels). But when the branching vessels become stiffer with increased elastic modulus, such changes in local reflection coefficient is rather moderate (Fig. 5.3.4). This indicates that junction geometry is more dominant in determining pulse transmission through vascular branching than elastic factors.

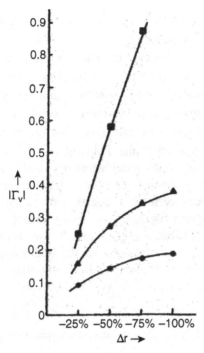

Fig. 5.3.3: Local reflection coefficient is plotted against the reduction in radius. Sharply increased reflection coefficient is associated with narrowing branching vessel lumen radius.

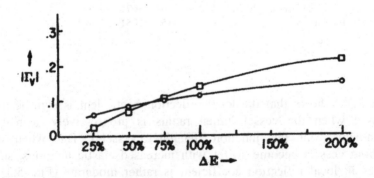

Fig. 5.3.4: Local reflection coefficient is plotted against the reduction in elastic modulus. Reflection is increased with increased branching vessel stiffness, but the increase is less pronounced as compared with corresponding percentage reduction in lumen radius.

5.4 Optimization Aspects Applicable to Vascular Branching

5.4.1 *Optimizing Vessel Radius and the Cube Law*

To overcome the resistance to blood flow, the power required will be inversely proportional to the fourth power of radius, or r^4, according to Poiseuille's law governing steady flow through a rigid cylindrical vessel (Fig. 5.4.1):

$$P_1 = R_s Q^2 \qquad (5.4.1)$$

where the Poiseuille resistance, R_s, to steady flow Q, is

$$R_s = \frac{8\eta l}{\pi r^4} \qquad (5.4.2)$$

where l is the length of the vessel along which blood flows. Thus, a larger vessel radius is more advantageous. This is because the flowing blood encounters a smaller resistance. However, a greater volume of blood is required for perfusion through a vessel with a larger radius, hence a greater demand on metabolic energy:

$$V = \pi r^2 l \qquad (5.4.3)$$

where V is the blood vessel volume.

The amount of volume flow, Q, is proportional to the square of the lumen radius, r^2, assuming the vessel is cylindrical:

$$Q = \pi r^2 v \qquad (5.4.4)$$

where v is linear blood flow velocity.

The optimal radius is therefore the one that can minimize the resistance to blood flow, as well as the power of expenditure. This can be formulated as:

$$P_o = k_1 \frac{1}{r^4} + k_2 r^2 \qquad (5.4.5)$$

where k_1 and k_2 are constants.

Differentiate P_o with respect to r, we have:

$$\frac{dP_o}{dr} = \frac{-4k_1}{r^5} + 2k_2 r = 0 \qquad (5.4.6)$$

Substituting equations (5.4.1) and (5.4.2) into (5.4.6), we obtain:

$$Q^2 = \frac{k_2 \pi}{16 \eta l} r^6 \qquad (5.4.7)$$

which gives an expression relating flow to the optimal vessel radius. We see that the flow is proportional to the cube of the vessel radius:

$$Q \propto r^3 \qquad (5.4.8)$$

This relation is the well-known "cube law". It is sometimes known as Murray's law. It states that in order to achieve a minimum amount of the rate of energy, the blood flow required to perfuse a blood vessel must be proportional to the cubic power of the radius. Controversy arises in the application of Murray's law. This stems from the fact that most of the resistance to blood flow are presented by small peripheral vessels (equation (5.4.2)), but that flow dominates in large vessels, such as the aorta. The applicability of the Murray's law therefore relies on where in the vasculature it is applied to.

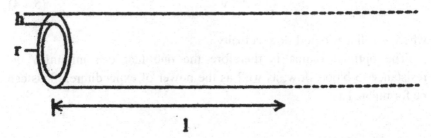

Fig. 5.4.1: A cylindrical blood vessel with radius r and length l.

Murray's (1926) minimum energy and Rosen's (1967) "Optimality Principles in Biology" have influenced earlier analysis of optimum branching. They both considered the use of a "cost function" which is commonly used in control systems engineering. The cost function considered is the sum of the rate of work done on the perfusing blood and the rate at which energy is utilized. This results in a cost function in terms of power associated with the flow-vessel interaction:

$$P_o = Q\Delta p + k(\pi r^2 l) \tag{5.4.9}$$

Where the first term is simply the rate of pressure-volume work and the second term is dependent on the volume of the vessel, assuming cylindrical in shape, with radius r and length, l (Fig. 5.4.1). Steady flow, Q, and pressure drop, Δp are considered here.

Power is the rate of energy use, i.e.

$$W = \int_0^T p(t)Q(t)dt \tag{5.4.10}$$

where p(t) and Q(t) are the pulsatile pressure and flow respectively and the instantaneous power is then

$$P_o = p(t)Q(t) \tag{5.4.11}$$

Equation (5.4.1) can be rewritten, employing Poiseuille's formula, as

$$P_v = (\frac{8\eta l}{\pi r^4})Q^2 + k(\pi r^2 l) \tag{5.4.12}$$

The optimal vascular system in this concept is plausible only when individual vessel segments are optimized. Minimum rate of work is obtained, by differentiating P_v with respect to r,

$$\frac{dP_v}{dr} = -\frac{32\eta l}{\pi r^5}Q^2 + 2k\pi r l \tag{5.4.13}$$

giving

$$r = \left(\frac{16\eta}{\pi^2 k}\right)^{1/6} Q^{1/3} \tag{5.4.14}$$

which is identical to eqn. (5.4.7), specifying the "cube-law" (eqn. (5.4.8)). For this radius, substituting into eqn. (5.4.12), the corresponding minimum rate of energy is

$$P_v = \frac{3k}{2}\pi r^2 l \tag{5.4.15}$$

Thus, the optimal radius for a blood vessel when the minimum rate of energy is required for steady flow is proportional to the 1/3 power of flow, Q.

5.4.2 *Optimizing Branching Radii and Angles*

Now consider a bifurcation with a mother vessel with length l_0 and radius r_0 that branches into two daughter vessels with lengths and radii of l_1, l_2 and r_1 and r_2, respectively, as shown in Fig. 5.4.2. It is assumed that the vessels are lying in the same plane.

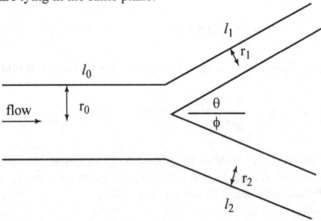

Fig. 5.4.2: Schematic drawing of a bifurcating vascular branching junction. A mother vessel branches into two daughter vessels. Lumen radius, length and bifurcation angles are shown.

We have for the cost function that assumes optimum rate of energy usage given by equation (5.4.15)

$$P_v = \frac{3k}{2}(\pi r_0^2 l_0 + \pi r_1^2 l_1 + \pi r_2^2 l_2) \tag{5.4.16}$$

The conservation of mass gives the equation of continuity of

$$Q_0 = Q_1 + Q_2 \tag{5.4.17}$$

which gives rise to the relation for the branching radii, from (5.4.6):

$$r_0^3 = r_1^3 + r_2^3 \tag{5.4.18}$$

which is again known as Murray's law or the "cube law for bifurcation".

Defining an area ratio as the sum of the daughter vessel lumen areas over the mother vessel lumen area, we have:

$$A_r = \frac{r_1^2 + r_2^2}{r_0^2} \tag{5.4.19}$$

For an equi-bifurcation, or that $r_1 = r_2$, we have

$$r_0^{3/2} = (2r_1^3)^{1/2} \tag{5.4.20}$$

Substitute, we have, for the area ratio:

$$A_r = 1.26 \tag{5.4.21}$$

When the angle of branching is involved, with half angles of branching of θ and φ, the optimum rate of energy is obtained when

$$r_0^2 = r_1^2 \cos\theta + r_2^2 \cos\varphi \tag{5.4.22}$$

Extensive data of vascular branches have been obtained by several investigators for vascular branches in different vascular beds (e.g. Li *et al.*, 1984; Schmidt-Shoenbein, 1986; Kassab *et al.*, 1993; Fung, 1995; Zamir, 2000). Data from pig coronary arteries by Kassab *et al.* (1993) show that Murray's law works very well in both control and hypertension hearts. A modified cost function is one that includes a metabolic constant k_m and takes into consideration the wall thickness of the vessel, h:

$$P_v = (\frac{8\eta l}{\pi r^4})Q^2 + k(\pi r^2 l) + k_m(2\pi r h l) \qquad (5.4.23)$$

This does not appear to differ significantly from Murray's formulation.

Chapter 6

The Venous System

6.1 The Reservoir Properties and Venous Return

6.1.1 *Venous Compliance and Reservoir Characteristics*

Veins are the principal conduits by which deoxygenated blood is returned to the heart, thus together with the arterial system, completing the closed-loop feature of the cardiovascular system. Blood from capillaries are returned through collecting venules to small veins and to large veins. Except the largest veins, i.e. vena cava, the great pulmonary veins and the smallest venules, veins have valves whose primary function is to facilitate the unidirectional return of blood to the heart and prevent backflow.

The reservoir properties of the veins can be easily appreciated, since more than 70% of the total blood volume of the systemic vascular system is contained in veins under normal conditions, as we have seen in Fig. 2.1.2. Hemodynamically speaking, this is because of the large compliance, due to a large incremental volume (dV) and small change in pulsatile distending pressure (dP), viz.

$$C = \frac{dV}{dP} \qquad (6.1.1)$$

The reservoir property can also be easily appreciated in the case of hemorrhage or blood loss events. Under such condition, venous blood volume, not arterial blood volume, decreases in order to maintain sufficient arterial perfusion pressure. This is accomplished by the

167

innervation of sympathetic fibers lining the venous walls, stimulation of which causes vasoconstriction, and the narrowing of lumen diameters, hence a reduction in volume of the venous reservoir. Thus, the interplay of reflex action and the volume adjustment, allow venous pressure also to be maintained. The volume loss is normally restored through fluid retention and replenishment. Fluid replenishment during hemorrhage is a topic of considerable clinical importance, particularly in reference to hemodilution (e.g. Kaya and Li, 2002; Pliskow *et al.*, 2016).

Venous pressures are generally low, seldom exceed 12 mm Hg, or 10% of the normal systolic pressure in arteries (120 mmHg). Veins have considerably smaller wall thickness-to-radius ratio (h/r) than corresponding arteries. This gives rise to the reservoir properties of the veins because of their distensibility. In comparison, the walls of veins are much thinner, with less smooth muscle cells, and are less stiff than arterial walls. The large diameter and low pressure of veins permits the venous system to function as a storage reservoir for blood. But the relatively weak wall also makes veins more easily torn under greater shear stress or pressure.

Veins acting as a storage reservoir of blood, also exhibit the function of blood distribution. Thus, they provide a critical element in blood volume control. For instance, in muscular parts of the body, such as upper and lower limbs, venous return is aided by the increase in venous tone so that the skeletal muscle pump increases venous pressure to ensure returning of blood to the heart. This is in addition to the peristaltic action of the veins and the one-way flow valves within the veins. The failure of the skeletal muscle contraction can lead to the common phenomenon of "venous pooling" of blood in the venous system of these limbs. Veins also play a major role in body organ temperature control through countercurrent exchanger mechanism. This latter is particularly effective in smaller vessels.

6.1.2 *Structural Properties of Veins*

Structurally speaking, veins and arteries have the same histological components as arteries, but with different contents and composition. The relatively thin wall of the veins, also contributes greatly to the large observed compliance. The collapsibility of the vein is due to several factors including: thin-walled vessel, large compliance, low transmural pressure. The latter is the principal controlling factor, as we shall see in the next section.

Despite the differences in structural and mechanical properties between arteries and veins, saphenous vein continues to be the most commonly utilized vessel in coronary artery bypass surgery. The difference in elastic properties between arteries and veins is well appreciated from their differences in distending pressure and wall structure.

As mentioned above, venous walls are much thinner than those of correspondingly sized arteries, and are truly thin-walled vessels, i.e. $h/r<1/10$. They contain much less smooth muscle and less elastic than arteries. Because of the collagen elastin composition, they exhibit less elastic recoil, but are easily stretched. Short-term venous blood redistribution can be accomplished by smooth muscle tone, or activation of sympathetic nerve fibers imbedded in the venous walls. Smooth muscle activation can alter the underlying elastic properties.

Veins are known to be non-circular in cross-section. Its collapsibility has been debated as to its inefficiency in metabolite transportation and blood flow. It has been shown that for an efficient fluid flow, the vessel ideally needs to be cylindrical. This implies a circular cross-sectional area. Veins however, often exhibit an elliptical cross-sectional area. With an eccentricity ratio of 2 (major axis diameter/minor axis diameter), the power required to deliver the same amount of blood is almost twice (125/64) that for a circular vessel lumen. In other words, for a given amount of power, the blood flow through an elliptical vessel lumen is about half (64/125) that of a circular lumen. However, this inefficiency is well made up by the presence of venous valves which arteries lack. These valves serve as auxiliary one-way facilitators that reduce backflow which are energetically wasteful.

6.1.3 *Venous Return*

The heart fills with blood during diastole. Thus, the amount of venous return and filling pressure are both important governing factors of adequate filling and subsequent ejection. Superior and inferior vena cava are the principal large veins that return blood to the heart. Being in the thorax, the intrathoracic pressure is also an importance consideration. A positive filling pressure must be maintained in these veins to facilitate venous return. This is necessarily so independent of body position, magnitude and distribution of blood volume. Maintaining this proper central venous pressure (CVP) requires the venous system to rapidly adjust to change in blood volume (BV) and its distribution. Since the vena cavae return blood to the right atrium, it is important that the venous pressure is slightly above the right atrial pressure. This is also necessary to prevent collapse when the difference of intravascular pressure (p_i) and extravascular pressure (p_e) becomes essentially zero or negative

$$\Delta p = p_i - p_e \qquad (6.1.2)$$

Right atrial pressure is often considered as the "preload" to the pumping function of the heart. It is also often referred to as the filling pressure. Normal filling pressure is typically below 12 mmHg. Extremely high right atrial or filling pressure thus can hinder venous return. In coronary heart diseased subjects, it is not unusual to find filling pressure that exceeds 30 mmHg.

During exercise, the increased cardiac output depends also on an increased amount of venous return to the heart. Reduced filling due to lower venous return can result in reduced stroke volume, reflected in the well-known Starling's law. It is recognized that increased sympathetic smooth muscle activation in the venous walls or venous tone in conjunction with compression of veins by surrounding skeletal muscles are important, together with the unidirectional venous valves, in returning blood towards the heart.

6.2 Pressure and Flow Waveforms in Veins

6.2.1 *The Normal Pressure and Flow Waveforms in Veins*

Since veins are the major conduits that return blood to the heart, their pressure and flow waveforms must be intimately related to cardiac function. This view has been deemed important particularly when considering large veins, such as the jugular vein, the main pulmonary vein and the vena cava. Veins are larger, but thinner, than their companion arteries. The relatively lower elastic modulus and greater compliance are reflected in the mechanical properties of the veins when stress-strain relations are examined. Since veins and arteries are normally structured in parallel and in close proximity to each other, there is usually cross-talk in pulsations, particularly the influence of arterial pressure oscillations on venous pulse waveform. This is seen in the jugular venous pulse, which is often compounded with the high pressure carotid artery pulse. The second major influence of the pulse waveform comes from cardiac chamber pressures, particularly that of the right and left atria. Thus, central venous pulses are important indicators of cardiac function.

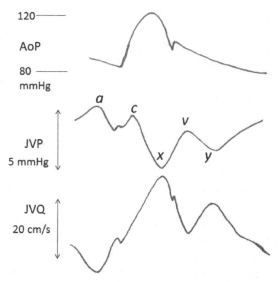

Fig. 6.2.1: Sketch of the jugular venous pressure (JVP) and flow velocity (JVQ) in relation to the ascending aortic pressure waveform (AoP). The characteristic a, c, v, x, y waves associated with JVP are seen. Note the striking difference in pressure amplitudes.

Unlike arterial pressure and flow waveforms, those of veins can vary considerably, subjecting to its collapsibility and external factors. Several features can be identified, however, from a typical venous pulse. Figure 6.2.1 illustrates the jugular pressure and flow waveforms when compared with the aortic pressure waveform. The a wave reflects right atria contraction. This is followed by the x decent or valley, due to atrial relaxation. The c wave is attributed to the carotid artery cross-talk or the systolic bulging of the tricuspid valve during the onset of ventricular systole. The v wave occurs during ventricular relaxation. The y decent or valley is during the onset of the rapid filling phase. These acxvy landmarks in jugular venous pressure waveform can be easily altered with small perturbations, and significantly so in diseased conditions.

The jugular venous waveform reflects events occurring in the right atrium and right ventricle. Frequently, landmarks on the recording of the phasic waveform of the jugular venous pulse are often similar to the pressure waveforms of the jugular vein, superior vena cava, and the right atrium.

The relation of atrial function and venous flow has been studied by some investigators. Goto *et al.* (1988) used laser Doppler velocimeter and an optical fiber to measure blood flow velocity in the small vein and artery of the left atrium of a dog. The vein velocity was characterized by a prominent atrial systolic flow. A considerable phase difference between arterial inflow and venous outflow was found and attributed to intravascular compliance properties.

6.2.2 *Respiration Effects on Venous Pressure and Flow Waveforms*

Because the major central veins are within the thorax, respiration can have a profound influence on the central venous pressure and flow waveforms. In addition, they modify the venous return to the heart. Moreno (1978) provided recordings of venous pressure and flow waveforms subjecting to such respiratory effects. In an awake, instrumented dog, the respiratory effect is well demonstrated when simultaneous measurements of pulmonary vein pressure and flow, vena caval flow, aortic and pulmonary aortic flows are recorded (Morgan *et al.*, 1966). This group of investigators found that vena cava flow reverses during atrial contraction. Additionally, the pulmonary vein pressure and flow peak in an almost out-of-phase manner (see also Fig. 6.2.1).

6.2.3 *Abnormal Venous Pressure and Flow Waveforms*

As mentioned earlier that central venous pulse reflects the conditions of the heart. Benchimol (1981) showed that there can be a prominent h wave, preceding the atrial contraction, associated with abnormal filling beyond the normally identifiable *acxvy* landmarks. Abnormal filling is particularly relevant in the analysis of venous pressure and flow waveforms.

Recordings of jugular pressure pulse often utilize tonometer, while the recording of jugular venous flow uses ultrasound Doppler velocity probe. The placement and angling of this transducer and the applied pressure are critical to the accuracy of the recorded signals. These are discussed in Chapter 8.

6.3 Modeling and Collapsible Vessel Properties

6.3.1 *Steady Flow in Collapsible Tubes*

That veins collapse is commonplace. The collapsibility is easily demonstrated by applying even a slight pressure over superficial veins, one can observe both venous pooling (bulging vein) and flow cessation due to occlusion. Transmural pressure is the difference between intravascular and extravascular or ambient pressure:

$$p_t = p_i - p_e \qquad (6.3.1)$$

We have seen that the veins have low pulse pressure oscillating with p_t close to zero.

The collapsible tube with flow is connected by rigid connections to two reservoirs. The tube is enclosed in a chamber, containing, say water with an adjustable external pressure p_e. Such a resistor is first used by Starling in his heart-lung machine a century ago (Knowlton and Starling, 1912). The flow in this tube is governed by the pressure differences, p_1-p_e and p_2-p_e. The amount of flow is dependent on the cross-section of the tube, and hence the transmural pressure. If the inlet pressure p_1 and the external pressure p_e were fixed, i.e. a constant p_1-p_e, then the flow velocity increases with decreasing p_2-p_e. But with this, the cross-sectional area decreases, hence the volume flow which is the product of velocity and cross-sectional area first increases, then becomes limited. This flow-limiting phenomenon is well illustrated by Holt (1941).

Assume laminar flow at a large Reynolds number so that Bernoulli's equation holds:

$$p_0 = p + \frac{1}{2}\rho v^2 \qquad (6.3.2)$$

where p is the static pressure and p_0 is the stagnation pressure and ρ is density of the fluid and v is flow velocity. The volume flow rate is obtained as the product of the cross-sectional area and the average velocity, i.e.

$$Q = Av = A\sqrt{\frac{2(p_0 - p)}{\rho}} = A\sqrt{\frac{2}{\rho}[(p_0 - p_e) - (p - p_e)]} \qquad (6.3.3)$$

A is the cross-sectional area which is a function of (p-p_e). Conservation of mass states that Q remains constant along the tube, despite that p varies with distance down the tube. If (p_0-p_e) is fixed, then the flow rate changes with (p-p_e):

$$\frac{dQ}{d(p - p_e)} = -\frac{A}{\rho v} + \left[\frac{p}{A}\frac{dA}{d(p - p_e)}\right]\frac{A}{\rho}v \qquad (6.3.4)$$

Pulse wave velocity can be derived with modification of the Moens-Korteweg formula. Area elasticity can be used instead of volume elasticity. Phase velocity of propagation in terms of pressure-cross-sectional area relation can be written as

$$c = \sqrt{\frac{A}{\rho}\frac{dp}{dA}} \qquad (6.3.5)$$

or

$$c^2 = \frac{A}{\rho} \frac{d(p - p_e)}{dA} \qquad (6.3.6)$$

Thus, equation (3) becomes:

$$\frac{dQ}{d(p - p_e)} = \frac{A}{\rho v}\left[(\frac{v}{c})^2 - 1\right] \qquad (6.3.7)$$

Thus, flow will increase with decreasing (p-p$_e$), only if v<c. Flow reaches its maximum and limitation occurs when v=c. If v>c, then a further decrease in (p-p$_e$) actually leads to a decrease in the flow. When the pulse wave velocity is low, as compared with flow velocity, the latter condition can occur. This v/c is known as the velocity fluctuation ratio or analogous to the Mach number.

Distensibility of the elastic tube is given as

$$D = \frac{1}{A} \frac{dA}{d(p - p_e)} \qquad (6.3.8)$$

6.3.2 *Flow Limitation and Model Experiments*

Holt's first such investigation has set the milestone for researchers on collapsible tube behavior and veins. His set-up is shown in Fig. 6.3.1. As above, flow Q through a segment of the collapsible tube is a function of the pressure just upstream to the collapsible segment, p1, the pressure just downstream to it, p2, and the external pressure within the enclosed chamber, pe. The experimental results for the Penrose tube are shown also in Fig. 6.3.1.

When the upstream pressure is greater than the downstream pressure (p1>p2) and the downstream pressure exceeds the external pressure, p2>pe, the vessel is simply open over its entire length. The slope of the p1-p2 vs. Q is determined by the flow resistance of the cylindrical tube. The more interesting result occurs when p2<pe, i.e. the tube no longer has a circular cross-section and is partially collapsed. Holt observed that flow to be constant in this range and described it as autoregulation, i.e. flow is now longer determined by the difference of upstream and

downstream pressures, p1-p2, but by p1-pe. Flow limitation is said to be reached at this point.

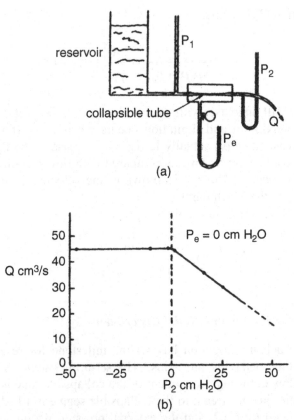

(a)

(b)

Fig. 6.3.1: (a) Flow in collapsible tube experimental set-up. The upstream and downstream pressures to the collapsible tube are p₁ and p₂, respectively. The external pressure is denoted by pₑ. (b) Flow (Q) as a function of downstream pressure (p₂), keeping pₑ and reservoir head constant. From Holt (1969).

Several investigators have giving terms to the phenomenon observed that when there is constant flow with downstream pressure varying (Holt's experiment) as "flow regulator" (Robard, 1963; Holt, 1969). While Permutt *et al.* (1962) attribute it to the "vascular waterfall" suggesting flow may be independent of downstream pressure. Conrad's detailed account used the tunnel diode analogy and suggested "negative impedance" between pressure drop across the collapsible tube and flow (Fig. 6.3.2).

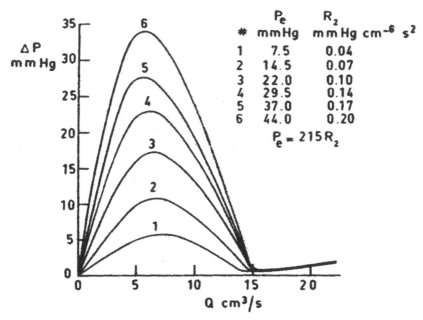

Fig. 6.3.2: Relationship of pressure gradient Δp (p₁-p₂) across the collapsible tube and flow (Q) with increasing (1 to 6) external pressure pₑ and nonlinear resistance, R₂. Notice the region when impedance is negative (decreasing Δp with increasing Q). From Conrad (1969).

Brower and Noordergaaf (1973) chose to consider the pressure drop across the collapsible tube as a function of flow and the difference between external pressure and downstream pressure as the primary determinants of pressure-flow relationship in a collapsible vessel, viz:

$$p_1 - p_2 = f(Q, p_e - p_2) \qquad (6.3.9)$$

They investigated this pressure drop (p₁-p₂) to flow relation as a function of various parameters that are derived from the fluid and the tube, i.e. elastic property of the vessel and its geometric dimension and the properties of the fluid. The resulting simple relation shows flow, Q, as a function of the pressure drop, p₁-p₂, with pₑ-p₂ as a parameter that was graded varying (Fig. 6.3.3). This figure resembles that of the transistor's voltage-current relationship. It can be seen here that the "negative impedance" concept suggested by Conrad does not exist here. Flow increases with pressure drop across the collapsible tube only within certain regime. At low pressure drop and low p_e-p_2, the relationship is more gradual and plateau is reached also gradually. At high pressure drop and high p_e-p_2, flow increases rapidly and reaching the plateau much faster. The plateau region reflects increases in flow that is independent of pressure drop Δp, across the collapsible vessel, p_1-p_2, and, the difference between external pressure and downstream pressure, p_e-p_2.

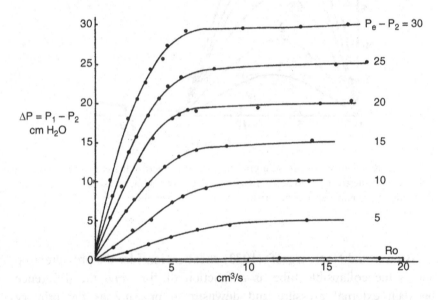

Fig. 6.3.3: Pressure gradient ($\Delta p = p_1$-p_2) and flow (Q) relation in a collapsible Penrose tube, while p_e-p_2 is varied. Ro is the equivalent Poiseuille resistance when tube is open.

In order to explain previous observations, Brower and Noordergraaf (1973) expressed the relation in terms of all the governing factors:

$$p_1 - p_2 = k_Q(p_e - p_2) \qquad (6.3.10)$$

This is true when

$$p_1 - p_2 \rangle RQ \qquad (6.3.11)$$

where k_Q is an empirical expression

$$k_Q = \frac{(Q/Q_c)}{[1+(Q/Q_c)^6]^{-1/6}}$$ (6.3.12)

where Q_c is the critical flow when the plateau is reached. It is an empirically derived function and is dependent on the values of p_e-p_2 only.

Otherwise, the whole relation reduces to that of a steady flow through the tube with circular cross-section:

$$p_1 - p_2 = RQ$$ (6.3.13)

An axially stretched Penrose tube showed no plateau (Brower and Noordergraaf, 1978) when Δp is plotted against flow.

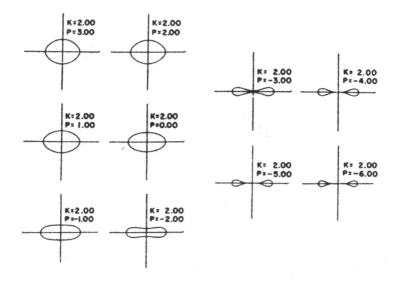

Fig. 6.3.4: Computed cross-sectional area shapes for a collapsible vessel with varying transmural pressure (p). Zero transmural pressure (p=0) is assumed to be an ellipse with eccentricity k=2.0.

Cross-sectional area in relation to transmural pressure in collapsible vessels has also been studied by several investigators. Kresch and Noordergrraaf (1972) computed the shapes of the tube cross-sectional areas for different eccentricity for negative transmural pressures, beginning with an ellipse cross-section when the transmural pressure is zero. The resulting shapes are shown in Fig. 6.3.4. Moreno *et al.*'s (1970) experimental findings seem to confirm these theoretically computed shapes.

6.3.3 *Pulse Wave Transmission Characteristics in Veins*

The low pulse pressure and collapsible nature of veins make pulse transmission measurements difficult. There are thus few studies. Anliker *et al.* (1969) utilized a method that ensure system linearity and avoid wave reflection effects. This latter is because wave reflection effects dominate at low frequencies (Chapter 4) and that the wave velocity is essentially constant, as is dynamic elastic modulus at high frequencies.

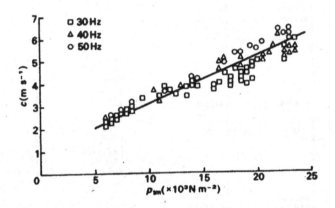

Fig. 6.3.5: Propagation velocity as a function of transmural pressure. Short trains of high frequency small amplitude sinusoidal pulse waves were imposed on the dog's abdominal vena cava. From Anliker *et al.* (1969).

They generated high frequency small amplitude sinusoidal pressure waveforms which were introduced into the abdominal vena cava of anesthetized dog or by means of an electromagnetic impactor attached to the veins outer wall. A dual-sensor catheter-tip transducer was inserted into the vein to measure pulse wave velocity from transit time delays, i.e. foot-to-foot velocity. Their results are shown in Fig. 6.3.5. It is clear from our earlier analysis that the pressure-dependence of compliance and pulse wave velocity are clearly seen with increasing transmural pressure.

Their results on attenuation showed that attenuation per wavelength is independent of frequency. Figure 6.3.6 shows that pulse wave amplitude declines with distance, described by:

$$a = a_0 e^{-kx / \lambda} \qquad (6.3.14)$$

where x is distance along the vessel, λ is wavelength of propagation, a is the amplitude and a_0 is the amplitude at x=0. The value of k for the vena cava of the dog is between 1.0 to 2.5, corresponding to attenuations of 63% to 92% per wavelength. This compares with 0.7 to 1.0 for the aorta. Thus, greater attenuation and slower pulse wave propagation velocity are found in the vena cava.

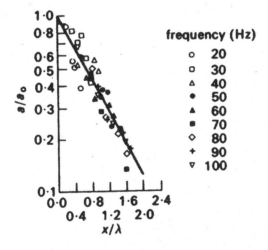

Fig. 6.3.6: Attenuation of short trains of high frequency small amplitude sinusoidal pulse waves were imposed on the dog's abdominal vena cava. Attenuation is represented by the amplitude ratio (a/a_0) as a function of changes in propagating distance as a fraction of wavelength (x/λ). From Anliker *et al.* (1969).

The attenuation was attributed to the viscosity of blood, the radial transmission to surrounding tissues and the viscoelastic properties of the walls. This latter is the predominating factor, as have been found for the systemic arteries by Li *et al.* (1981). That the attenuation per wavelength is practically independent of frequency suggest that the energy dissipation is independent of strain rate. A point of criticism arises as frequencies of 20-100 Hz was used in the study by Anliker *et al.*, much higher than the highest significant component of natural pulse pressure and flow waveforms.

Pulse wave velocity as seen from the above experimental measurements, is significantly lower in veins than in corresponding size arteries. This can be measured as foot-to-foot velocity or can be readily estimated from the Moens-Korteweg formula.

But with the changing cross-sectional area and the transmural pressure, pulse wave velocity is seen to be dependent on both vessel compliance and frequency. Brower and Scholten (1975) demonstrated this latter in a collapsible Penrose tube, while Anliker *et al.* (1969) measured this in dog veins. The former was analytically derived by Kresch and Noordergraaf (1969) for the case of uniform collapse tube:

$$c = \sqrt{\frac{A}{\rho(dA/dp)}} k_v \qquad (6.3.15)$$

where

$$k_v = [1 - \frac{2J_1(\sqrt{j\omega k_A})}{jwk_A J_0(\sqrt{j\omega k_A})}] \qquad (6.3.16)$$

$$k_A = \frac{\rho A}{\pi \eta k} \qquad (6.3.17)$$

Where J_0 and J_1 are Bessel function of the zeroth and first order and A is the cross-sectional area, dA/dp is the distensibility of a circular tube with the same cross-sectional area, κ is the shape factor which equals 1.0 for a circular vessel and 2.0 for a collapsed vessel, ρ and η are the density and viscosity of the fluid. Wave velocity is dependent on shape is observed by Bailie (1972). Thus, in this formulation the phase velocity is frequency dependent and cross-sectional area dependent.

Chapter 7

The Microcirculation

7.1 Structure of the Microcirculation

7.1.1 *Functional Organization of the Microvasculature*

The function of the cardiovascular system is to provide a homeostatic environment for the cells of the organism. The exchange of the essential nutrients and gaseous materials occurs in the microcirculation at the level of the capillaries. These microvessels are of extreme importance for the maintenance of a balanced constant cellular environment. Capillaries and venules are known as exchange vessels where the interchange between the contents in these walls and the interstitial space occur across their walls.

The microcirculation can be described in terms of a network such as that shown in Fig. 7.1.1. It consists of an arteriole and its major branches, the metarterioles. The metarterioles lead to the true capillaries via a precapillary sphincter. The capillaries gather to form small venules, which in turn become the collecting venules. There can be vessels going directly from the metarterioles to the venules without supplying capillary beds. These vessels form arteriovenous (A-V) shunts and are called arteriovenous capillaries. The thickness of the wall and endothelium of these structures and the proportionate amounts of the various vascular wall components are shown in Chapter 2. The capillary and venule have very thin walls. The capillary, as mentioned before, lacks smooth muscle and only has a layer of endothelium. The smooth muscle and elastic tissue are present in greater amounts in vessels having vasoactive capabilities, such as arterioles. This is also the site of greatest drop in mean blood pressure in the systemic circulation. For this reason, arterioles are the principal contributors to peripheral vascular resistance that can effectively alter cardiac output. Thus, mean blood pressure, cardiac output and peripheral resistance bear a close relation in the control and regulation of circulatory function.

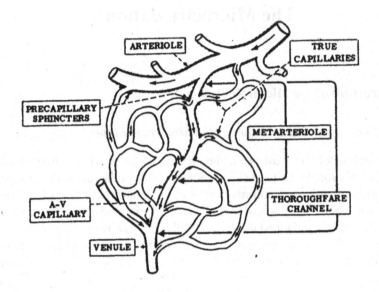

Fig. 7.1.1: A network of microcirculatory unit, illustrating the constituent components.

The structural components of the microcirculation are classified into resistance, exchange, shunt, and capacitance vessels. The resistance vessels, comprising the arterioles, metarterioles, and precapillary sphincters, serve primarily to decrease the arterial pressure to the levels of the capillaries to facilitate effective exchange.

Differences in microvascular behavior are attributed to the differences in the overall function of the body organ in which these microvessels exist. Thus, flow in the microvessels of the brain differs from that in the heart or the lungs. Some capillaries are fed by the arterioles and collected by the venules, but others can bypass the capillaries and connected directly to either small artery to a small vein. These latter are known as anastomoses which serve to control flow and certain transport processes. It is well-known in the countercurrent mechanism for body temperature control, the small arteries and veins run parallel and frequently adjacent to each other, while branching arterioles and venules are close to 90°. Capillaries, in general, are running parallel next to perfusing muscle or tissues. These are well illustrated by the photomicrographs of Smaje *et al.* (1970) in the cremaster muscle of the rat (Fig. 7.1.2) and also by Zwifach *et al.* (1974) in the cat omentum (Fig. 7.1.3).

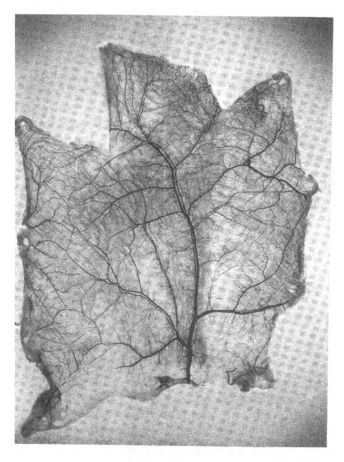

Fig. 7.1.2: Photomicrograph of rat cremaster muscle showing pattern of vascular structure. Y-shaped and T-shaped branching junctions are common, in addition to cross-connections of the vessels. From Smaje *et al.* (1970).

A bat (a flying mammal) wing and the mesenteric bed of a small mammal are popular preparations for studying blood flow in the microcirculation. The flow into the capillaries has been shown to remain pulsatile or intermittent in nature (e.g. Zweifach, 1974). It has also been shown that the rhythmic vasomotor activity of the precapillary sphincters is responsible for the observed intermittency. The sphincters may also exhibit constriction and dilation in response to changes in local metabolites, chemicals, or sympathetic stimuli. Together with the arterioles, the precapillary sphincters serve to adjust the amount of blood flow to meet the demands in tissues.

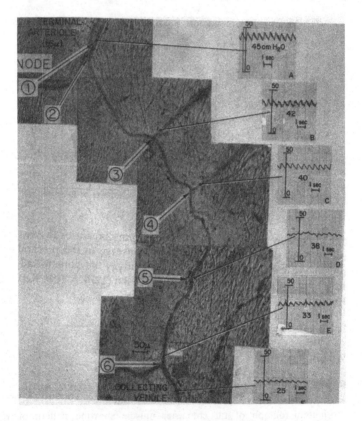

Fig. 7.1.3: Photomicrographic reconstruction of the microcirculation from a terminal arteriole through capillaries to a collecting venule. The flow into the capillaries remains pulsatile or intermittent. Direct pulsatile pressure recordings are shown. From Zweifach (1974).

If we compare the size of red cells from various mammals, we find the perhaps surprising fact that their diameters seem to be rather uniform and independent of mammalian body size (Li, 1996). This is summarized in Table 7.1.1. Data from more than one hundred mammalian species show that the red blood cells are of similar size and that there is no single mammal has a red blood cell diameter over 10 μm. This suggests the structural sizes of the capillaries are in the same order of magnitude in these mammals. It should be noted however, that the structures and functions of the endothelial cells lining the capillaries may differ, depending on the microvascular bed of a particular organ they serve. In addition, the topological branching structures of the different microvascular beds are unique for each organ. For instance, the pulmonary microcirculation has an entirely different vascular tree structure as compared to the coronary microcirculation, or that of the cerebral microcirculation.

Table 7.1.1: Diameters of red blood cells (RBC) of some mammalian species.

Species	Body weight (kg)	RBC Diameter (μm)
Shrew	.01	7.5
Mouse	.20	6.6
Rat	.50	6.8
Dog	20	7.1
Man	70	7.5
Cattle	300	5.9
Horse	400	5.5
Elephant	2000	9.2

Unlike the capillaries, the arteriole (10-125 μm) has smooth muscle cell layers in its wall with the nerve connection to its outermost layer. Even the terminal arteriole still has a single layer of smooth muscle cells. A meta-arteriole has a discontinuous layer of smooth muscle cells. Pre-capillary sphincter is the last smooth muscle cell at the end of terminal arterioles. Similarly, there are post-capillary venules, and collecting venules (10-50 μm) and small collecting veins which already has intima endothelial layer, the media with smooth muscle layers.

7.1.2 *The Capillary Circulation*

The extensiveness of the organizational structure of the network of capillaries is necessary for efficient cellular transport and diffusion processes to take place. These processes are slow in comparison to blood perfusion. For this reason, a capillary is normally in the neighborhood and within reach to any single cell at a distance of about three to four cells apart. A given capillary can have a length of about 1 mm and a diameter of 5-10 μm.

Two principal types of capillaries are found. The true capillaries have no vascular smooth muscle and form network with other capillaries. The arterio-venous or A-V capillaries have some amount of smooth muscle and are directly connected to muscular arterioles and small venules. Phasic flow patterns are determined by the vasomotion, attributed to the small arterioles, the A-V capillaries, the precapillary sphincters. These latter gives rise to the constant dilation and constriction that modulate the flowing blood. Local control dominates, as the precapillary sphincters do not have nerve connections. The true capillary walls are without connective tissue and smooth muscle and consist of a single layer of endothelial cells surrounded by a basement membrane of collagen and mucopolysaccharides.

Differences in capillary endothelium structure give rise to different capillary function in different tissues. These can continuous capillaries, fenestrated capillaries or sinusoid capillaries. In a continuous capillary 4 nm clefts, a complete basement membrane and numerous vesicles can be seen. The fenestrated capillary is one with pores through a thin portion of the wall, few vesicles and a complete basement membrane, while a sinusoidal capillary has large para-cellular gaps extending through the discontinuous basement membrane. Because of the structural differences, the continuous capillary has been found to be the least permeable, while the sinusoidal capillary, the most permeable. Continuous capillaries are found, for instances, in muscle, nervous tissue and the lungs. The fenestrated capillaries are found, for example, in intestines. The sinusoidal capillaries are located, for instances, in the liver, adrenal cortex and bone marrow.

Nutrients and formed substances can move across the wall of continuous capillaries either through or between the endothelial cells. Lipid-soluble substances diffuse through the cell membrane. Water and ions diffuse through the water-filled clefts between cells. There are transport mechanisms that allow glucose, some amino acids and macromolecules to move across some capillary walls. Some of thee mechanisms have not been elucidated. One such mechanism is through vesicle-mediated transport process.

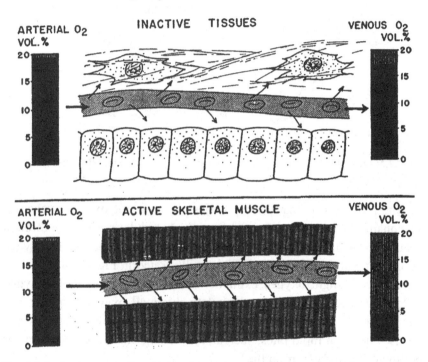

Fig. 7.1.4: Oxygen extraction in inactive skin tissue (top) and active skeletal muscle tissue (bottom). From Rushmer (1972).

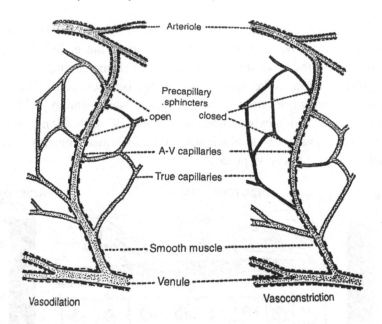

Fig. 7.1.5: Illustration of the vasomotion in a capillary network. From Rushmer (1972).

The primary role that the capillaries play is in the oxygen exchange. The quantity of oxygen extracted from the blood during its flow through capillaries is determined by the relationship between the rate of oxygen utilization and the blood flow. This is illustrated in Fig. 7.1.4. The top figure shows slight oxygen extraction and small arterio-venous oxygen differences occur in tissues with relatively small oxygen requirements and active blood, such as skin. The bottom figure shows tissues which release energy at rapid rates, such as contracting muscle, extract a major portion of the oxygen from the blood.

As we mentioned earlier, capillaries in some tissues may consist of arterio-venous (A-V) capillaries known as thoroughfare channels and true capillaries. The blood flow through different portions of the capillary bed is affected by contraction and relaxation of smooth muscle in the arterioles, A-V capillaries and precapillary sphincters. Phasic changes in these regions produce cyclic alterations in the amount and distribution of blood flow through the various capillaries. This is known as the vascular vasomotion (Fig. 7.1.5).

7.2 Pressure-Flow Relation and Microcirculatory Mechanics

7.2.1 *Flow-Related Mechanical Characteristics of the Microcirculation*

Pressure, flow and forces are drastically smaller in the microcirculation as opposed to the macrocirculation. We know that the Reynolds number as defined by

$$R_e = \frac{\rho v d}{\eta} \qquad (7.2.1)$$

is very small as compared to an artery. For instance, the Reynolds number may be 0.03 for a 100 μm arteriole. With even smaller diameter and blood velocity, the Reynolds number is at least an order smaller in the capillary.

Steady flow is assumed in many hemodynamic and rheological studies. This is because the Womersley's number (see also 4.5.28), defined as

$$\alpha_W = r\sqrt{\frac{\omega \rho}{\eta}} \qquad (7.2.2)$$

is very small. Womersley's number can be viewed as the ratio of oscillatory flow to steady flow. When α_W approaches zero, the approximation of a steady flow is a reasonable one.

In relation to entry length, it is now small compared with the diameter of the microvessels. Thus, the flow becomes fully developed towards a parabolic profile, despite the relatively short length of the vessels.

The Newtonian fluid aspect needs to be carefully addressed. The blood and its formed elements now contribute more to the abnormality of the viscosity. The well-known Fahraeus-Lindqvist effect explains the decreasing blood viscosity in very small vessels. Nevertheless, the Poiseuille's equation has been viewed as important in the microcirculation, in that the flow is determined by the driving force of the pressure gradient and the resisting force of viscosity.

$$Q = \frac{\pi r^4}{8\eta l} \Delta p \qquad (7.2.3)$$

Although remaining pulsatile, the flow in the capillaries is intermittent at best. A single arteriole branches into several and sometimes 15 or so capillaries. The branching phenomena and optimization aspect we discussed in Chapter 5, now needs to incorporate considerably more local control aspects, in terms of exchange between the capillaries and its surrounding tissues, as well as the vasomotion due to smooth muscle tone in the arterioles.

The flow into the capillaries has been shown to remain pulsatile or intermittent in nature. It has also been shown that the rhythmic vasomotor activity of the precapillary sphincters is responsible for the observed intermittency. The sphincters may also exhibit constriction and dilation in response to changes in local metabolites, chemicals, or sympathetic stimuli. Together with the arterioles, the precapillary sphincters serve to adjust the amount of blood flow to meet the demands in tissues.

Starling's hypothesis describes the filtration and absorption of fluid across capillary walls. The capillary wall is known to consist of endothelium with a basement membrane that is highly permeable to allow fluid exchange. Several factors govern such exchange: (1) hydrostatic capillary blood pressure, p_c, (2) osmotic pressure of plasma proteins, π_c, (3) hydrostatic interstitial fluid pressure, p_i and (4) osmotic pressure, π_i, of the proteins in the interstitial fluid. They define the Starling's hypothesis:

$$p_c - p_i = \pi_c - \pi_i \qquad (7.2.4)$$

under equilibrium. In other words, the difference in fluid pressure in the capillary and the surrounding interstitial tissue equals the difference in osmotic pressure between the capillary blood and the extravascular fluid.

Depending on the physiological demand, the microcirculatory system adjusts itself rapidly and efficiently. For this reason, the trans-capillary flow is given by a modification of eqn. (7.2.4) to:

$$Q = k_c A(p_c - p_i - \pi_c + \pi_i) \tag{7.2.5}$$

where k_c is capillary permeability, often referred to as filtration constant, and A is the cross-sectional area available for the exchange. Several methods are available to measure this flow, including the micro-occlusion and electro-optical techniques and the use of optical dye. Capillary permeability is in the order of $3 \cdot 10^9$ $g^{-1}cm^2s$. Fenestrated capillaries have higher kc than continuous capillaries. Increased capillary permeability is one of the many processes observed during inflammation.

7.2.2 Some Pressure-Related Mechanical Characteristics of the Microcirculation

Pressure measurement techniques in the microvessels were mostly based on the method originally designed by Wiederhielm *et al.* (1964). Zweifach and colleagues have refined the technique and performed extensive measurements (e.g. Zweifach, 1974 and Zweifach and Lipowsky, 1977). Figure 7.2.1 illustrates such an intravascular measurement of pressure and velocity in a cat mesentery microvascular bed. Arterial to venous distribution of the pressure and velocity is shown. Pressure dropped rapidly in small arterioles, but more gradually in the capillaries. The velocity drop parallels the velocity in the arterioles, not so on the venous side.

The pressure gradient, $\Delta p / \Delta z$ or dp/dL can be measured by the micro-occlusion technique. Here, two pressure probes are inserted into two side branches of a given vessel and flow is occluded in these side branches. The two pressure readings divided by the distance between the two measurement sites gives the pressure gradient.

Lee and Schmid-Shonbein (1995) have estimated distensibility of capillaries in skeletal muscles based on the pressure-area relation (see Chapter 2). They made a comparison of capillary distensibility when the fascia of the skeletal muscle is tact or removed (Fig. 7.2.2). It is interesting to note that the capillary distensibility is retained even when the fascia is intact for positive transmural pressures. However, the greater distensibility when fascia is removed case suggests that skeletal muscle contraction can influence capillary distensibility. The consequence is a reduction of the distensibility during contraction.

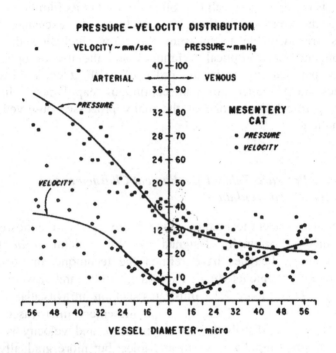

Fig. 7.2.1: Illustration of arterial to venous distribution of intravascular pressure and velocity in the cat mesentery as a function of microvessel diameters. Solid lines are fitted curves. From Zweifach and Lipowsky (1977).

The circumferential stress-strain relation of microvessels follow the curvilinear relations found arteries and veins, though to a greatly different extent. The circumferential stress-strain relation of isolated capillary blood vessels in gracilis muscle of Sprague-Dawley rats with fascia removed is shown in Fig. 7.2.3. Here, the capillary wall is not in contact with muscle fibers. The assumption is made that all the circumferential tension is carried by the basement membrane.

It should be noted here that the diameters of microvascular vessels change continuously throughout the cardiac cycle. Thus, the compliance change must follow the nonlinear behavior as we have shown earlier for the arteries. In other words, the compliance is pressure-dependent

(Chapter 4), thus time-varying. The measurements of diameters of subendocardial arterioles and subendocardial venules by Kajiya and his colleagues (Yada *et al.*, 1993) support this conclusion (Fig. 7.2.4).

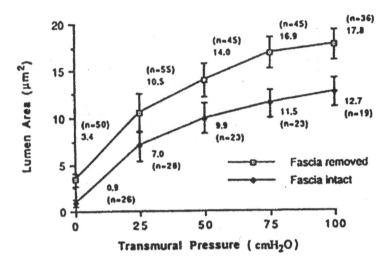

Fig. 7.2.2: Measurement of capillary distensibility in terms of lumen area and transmural pressure when fascia is either left intact or removed. From Lee and Schmid-Schonbein, (1995).

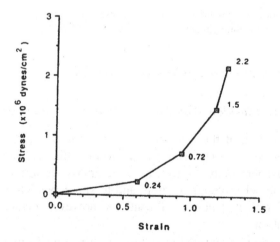

Fig. 7.2.3: Circumferential stress-strain relation of isolated capillary blood vessels. From Lee and Schmid-Schonbein (1995).

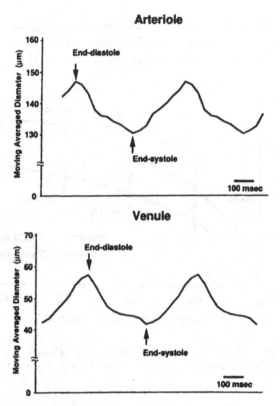

Fig. 7.2.4: Continuous variations of the diameters of a subendocardial arteriole and a subendocardial venule throughout the cardiac cycle. From Yada *et al.* (1993).

7.3 Pulse Transmission and Modeling Aspects

7.3.1 *Pressure and Flow Waveforms in Arterioles and Capillaries*

Pulses, originating at the left ventricle, are modified as they propagate toward the periphery. This is attributed to the effects of blood viscosity, to arterial viscoelasticity, as well as to geometry, resulting in frequency dispersion and selective attenuation, and to site dependent summation of incident and reflected pulses. Pulsations, however, persist even in the microcirculation.

Quantification of peripheral resistance has long been an interest to both researchers and clinicians. Since the largest mean pressure drop occur in the arteriolar beds. These latter have been suggested to be the principal contributor mostly to the total peripheral resistance.

It has been presumed for decades that flow in the microcirculation, particularly in the arterioles and capillaries, is entirely steady flow. Consequently, Poiseuille's formula has been applied. Poiseuille in 1841 arrived at an empirical relationship relating pressure drop Δp to steady flow (Q) in a cylindrical vessel with diameter D and length l. Thus, the amount of steady flow through a blood vessel is proportional to the pressure drop and the fourth power of the diameter. Independently, Hagen had performed numerous experiments and, at about the same time, arrived at a similar expression. This formula was later modified to the presently known Hagen-Poiseuille equation, or simply, the Poiseuille's law:

$$\overline{Q} = \frac{\pi r^4}{8\eta l} \Delta p \qquad (7.3.1)$$

Although credit has been given fully to Poiseuille, it was Hagenbach (1860) who came up with an exact relation relating steady flow to the fluid viscosity η, and the pressure gradient,

$$Q = -\frac{\pi r^4}{8\eta} \frac{dp}{dz} \qquad (7.3.2)$$

Pressure gradient in the Poiseuille's law is simply $\Delta p / \Delta z$ or $\Delta p / l$. Poiseuille resistance to steady flow is therefore:

$$R_s = \frac{8\eta l}{\pi r^4} \qquad (7.3.3)$$

Steady flow was assumed because of the belief that small peripheral vessels are resistance vessels, preventing pulsations from occurring.

As mentioned above, the largest mean pressure drop occurs in small arterioles. Referring back to Chapter 2 regarding the structure of the vascular walls, we see that this is also where smooth muscle tends to exert its influence. Thus, accompanying the smooth muscle (Somlyo and Somlyo, 1968) activation, is a change in vessel lumen radius. Since flow varies by the fourth power of radius, a small change in radius can amount to a large alteration in flow. Thus, the peripheral resistance can alter central arterial flow, hence cardiac output.

It is now known that pulsatile ejection by the ventricle requires only about 10% additional energy for the same stroke volume compared to constant outflow. This minimal additional energy associated with pulsatile ventricular ejection reflects the compliant properties of the receiving arterial tree, mostly due to large arteries.

An appreciable fraction of the energy in the pressure and flow pulses generated by the heart reaches the capillaries in pulsatile form. This has been demonstrated experimentally by, for instance, Wiederhelm *et al.* (1964), in frog's mesentery, Intaglietta *et al.* (1970, 1971) in cat omentum, Zweifach (1974), Zweifach and Lipowsky (1977) and Smaje *et al.* (1980). It has been postulated that pulsations are necessary to attain optimal organ function. Steady perfusion could impair organ function (Wilkins *et al.*, 1967; Jacobs *et al.*, 1969; Arnzelius, 1976). Direct recording of pressure obtained by Zweifach (1974) suggests that in the terminal arteriole, the pulse pressure is still large, about 15 mmHg, with a mean pressure of about 60 mmHg. Intaglietta *et al.* (1970) provided pulsatile velocity data. Mean velocities in the microcirculation are in the centimeters per second range, as measured by electro-optical methods.

7.3.2 Pulse Transmission Characteristics in the Microcirculation

The steady flow concept assumed for the microcirculation is in accordance with the windkessel theory that peripheral vessels act as stiff tubes. This would protect the small vessels against sudden surges in flow and rapid changes in pressure.

With the advent of new technology, particularly the servo-controlled micropipette device for pressure measurement and electro-optical methods, such as laser Doppler velocimeter, for velocity recording, studies of the pulse transmission in arterioles and capillaries became feasible. Although significantly damped, pressure and flow pulses generated by the heart persist into these vessels.

Li *et al.* (1980) first provided analytical expressions to predict pulse wave velocity and attenuation in the microcirculation. Linearized pulse transmission theory was utilized. Subsequently, the same group at Penn led by Noordergraaf computed the pulse transmission from the left ventricle to the human index finger vessel (Salotto *et al.*, 1986, Fig. 7.3.1). Their computation was based on Westerhof's viscoelastic tube theory, with complex elastic modulus.

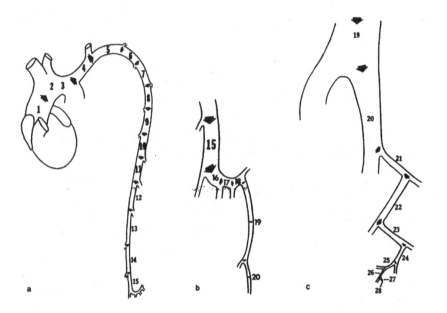

Fig. 7.3.1: Schematic illustration of the pulse transmission path from the ascending aorta (a, segment 1) to the index finger artery (c, segment 28). Such segmental approach allows each arterial segment's mechanical and geometrical properties, as well as propagation characteristics to be clearly defined.

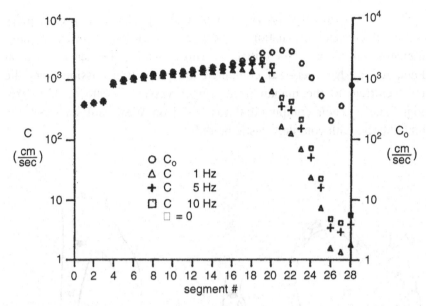

Fig. 7.3.2: Pulse wave velocity at different frequencies shown plotted as a function of transmission site from the ascending aorta to the index finger artery.

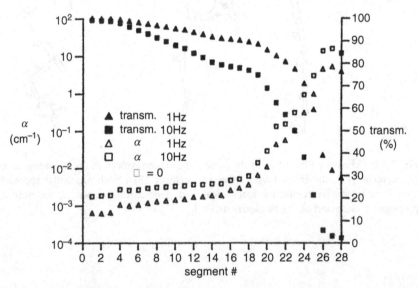

Fig. 7.3.3: Attenuation coefficient and percentage transmission at different frequencies (1 Hz and 10 Hz) shown plotted as a function of transmission site from the ascending aorta to the index finger artery.

The results show wave velocity of a few centimeters per second and attenuation of about 30 percent at I Hz in large arterioles. With increasing frequencies, the attenuation become substantial and pulse transmission is greatly reduced at 10 Hz. These are shown in Figs. 7.3.2 and 7.3.3. This explains in parts why the observed pressure and flow waveforms, though pulsatile, are becoming more sinusoidal in the microcirculation, as higher frequency component are damped out.

A wave speed of 7.2 cm/s in the capillary with an exponential attenuation of 83%/cm was calculated by Caro *et al.* (1978). Estimated phase velocity from Intaglietta *et al.*'s (1971) data would give 7-10 cm/s, in general agreement. They also gave an analytical expression for the propagation speed in the case of a sinusoidal pulse propagating through an elastic vessel, assuming blood is Newtonian:

$$c = \frac{1}{4} d \sqrt{\frac{\omega}{\eta D}} \tag{7.3.4}$$

where d is capillary diameter and D is the distensibility. Since blood viscosity appears to decrease when measured in capillary tubes of decreasing diameter, blood, in fact, is non-Newtonian. This is recognized as the Fahraeus-Lindqvist effect.

7.3.3 Modeling Aspects of the Microcirculation

Modeling of any microvascular bed has been a challenge, particularly when validation of predicted phenomena is concerned. A complete study requires not only the stringent measurement techniques, but also the understanding of the complexity of the underlying system properties.

Mayrovitz (1975, 1976) and Noordergraaf (1978) provided an analysis of a model of the microcirculatory dynamics. The bat wing was selected for the ease of accessibility and measurements of the microvascular bed parameters. A distributed model was developed based on the wing's vascular anatomy. The topology of this model is shown in Fig. 7.3.4 which includes a perfusing artery, arterioles and collecting venules and a vein, as well as capillaries, precapillary sphincter.

Geometric dimensions of the branching structure are also shown in the table. Poiseuille formula was utilized for describing small vessel pressure-flow relationship. Pressure distribution along the vascular bed and its change due to diameter alteration of fourth order branching vessels are shown in Fig. 7.3.5 during control, simulated contraction and vasodilation. Experimental results provide a validation that the model predicted pressure distributions are reasonably accurate.

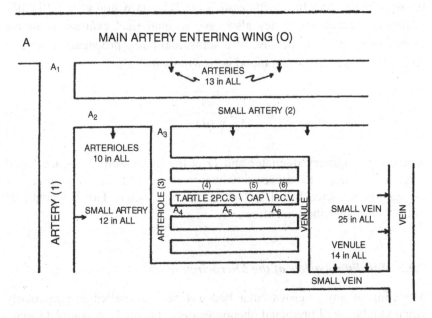

Fig. 7.3.4: Topological model of the microvascular bed of the bat wing. One pathway for a main artery to a vein is displayed. The branching order is numbered and the particular sites are denoted by A_1-A_6. Terminal arteriole (T. ARTLE), precapillary sphincter (P.C.S.), CAP (capillary) and post-capillary venule (P.C.V.) are also marked. Corresponding geometric dimensions are also shown in the table. From Mayrovitz (1976).

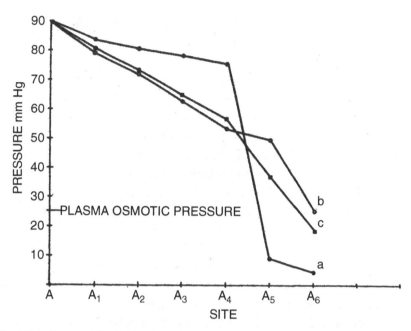

Fig. 7.3.5: Pressure distribution along the vascular bed and its change due to diameter alteration of fourth order branching vessels during control (c), simulated contraction (a) and dilation (b).

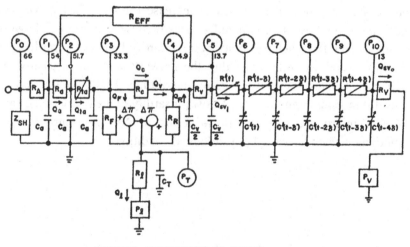

DETAILED MICROVASCULAR MODEL

Fig. 7.3.6: A dynamic microcirculatory model. P=pressure, Q=flow, R=resistance, C=compliance, $\Delta\pi$=osmotic pressure difference across the capillary wall.

A dynamic model was later developed by the same group that included resistance and capacitance, as well as time-varying compliance properties. The model shown in Fig. 7.3.6 also provided description of vasomotion, capillary filtration and re-absorption processes.

Hemodynamic pulsatility has long been reported to regulate microcirculatory function, as pulsatile perfusion has been shown to be more beneficial than steady flow to organ vascular beds, such as the cerebral and the renal. We recently quantitatively assessed the impact of flow pulsatility on the microvasculature (Wang *et al.*, 2017). In this, a mathematical model was first developed to simulate the regulation of NO production by pulsatile flow in the microcirculation. Pertinent parameters such as shear stress and pressure pulsatility were selected as regulators of endothelial NO production and NO-dependent vessel dilation as feedback to control microvascular hemodynamics. The model was then applied to a real experimentally obtained microvascular network of the rat mesentery consisting of 546 microvessels. As compared to steady flow conditions, pulsatile flow increased the average NO concentration in arterioles from 256.8 ± 93.1 nM to 274.8 ± 101.1 nM ($P < 0.001$), with a corresponding increase in vessel dilation by approximately 7% from $27.5 \pm 10.6\%$ to $29.4 \pm 11.4\%$ ($P < 0.001$). In contrast, NO concentration and vessel size showed a far lesser increase (about 1.7%) in venules under pulsatile flow as compared to steady flow conditions. Network perfusion and flow heterogeneity were improved under pulsatile flow conditions, and vasodilation within the network was more sensitive to heart rate changes than pulse pressure amplitude. This model proved to be useful in simulating the role of flow pulsatility in the regulation of any complex microvascular network in terms of NO concentration and hemodynamics under varied physiological conditions.

Chapter 8

Hemodynamic Measurements: Invasive and Noninvasive Monitoring

8.1 Catheterization for Blood Pressure Measurement

8.1.1 *Fluid-filled Blood Pressure Measurement Systems*

The combination of a fluid-filled catheter and a pressure transducer continues to be the most commonly used measurement system for in-vivo recording of pulsatile blood pressure waveforms. This blood pressure measurement system can be applied to cardiac chambers, major arteries and veins, as well as smaller (~1 mm) vessels of the circulation. This is because of the long, well-established and improved catheterization techniques in combination with angiographic imaging modalities in clinical catheterization laboratories. The catheter system has the added advantage of the ease of injecting radio-opaque dyes for visualization of the vasculature, as well as administering therapeutic drugs. Balloon catheter for angioplasty and vascular stent applications and micro-pore catheter for local intravascular drug delivery have also become popular. The more recent multi-lumen, multi-functional catheters include thermodilution, as well as the addition of electrodes for either atrial or ventricular pacing capabilities. These technological advances have promoted the popularity of interventional cardiology.

Forssmann and Cournand, who shared the 1956 Nobel Prize in Medicine with Richards, are the original inventors who decades earlier first recorded blood pressure waveforms in peripheral arteries and cardiac chambers. The catheter has the flexibility and maneuverability that allows accessibility to different parts of the circulation. There are instances, where a combination of a hypodermic needle and a pressure transducer suffices, particularly when the blood vessel is superficial or under intra-operative conditions. Brachial, radial or femoral arteries are common superficial sites for pressure measurements with needle-transducer systems. Left ventricular chamber pressure measurement with direct apex insertion of a needle is also common under open chest conditions.

Right heart catheterization was a newer development introduced in 1970 with the Swan-Ganz catheter. This is a balloon-tipped catheter introduced through a vein, such as the jugular, subclavian or femoral, to allow blood returning to the right heart pushing the balloon to where measurement is desired. This flow-directed catheter thus allows blood pressure measurements en route, i.e. of venous pressure, right atrial pressure, right ventricular pressure, pulmonary aortic pressure and that in smaller pulmonary vasculature for right heart diagnosis. It has an advantage that imaging is not required.

In evaluating accuracy of fluid-filled blood pressure measurement systems, techniques used in engineering is often employed. The performance of a needle-pressure transducer system can be evaluated through basic mechanical and electrical modeling. The simplest representation of the system is an undamped spring-mass system of natural frequency:

$$f_n = \frac{1}{2\pi}\sqrt{\frac{\pi r^2}{\rho l} \cdot \frac{dp}{dV}} \qquad (8.1.1)$$

where r is the internal lumen radius of the needle, l is the length of the needle and ρ is the fluid density. Typically the needle and pressure transducer dome are filled with saline. This provides the required fluid coupling that is necessary when the needle is inserted into an artery which is filled with blood. Heparin is often added to prevent blood clotting in the catheter. Blood pressure pulsation is transmitted via fluid coupling resulting in the movement of the pressure transducer diaphragm (stainless steel). The greater the amount of fluid, the greater is the fluid movement or inertia. Thus, the inertia is represented by

$$L = \frac{\rho l}{\pi r^2} \qquad (8.1.2)$$

The compliance of the pressure transducer is determined by the movement of the stainless steel diaphragm within the fluid-filled transducer dome. Compliance which is defined as volume displacement per unit distending pressure, is the inverse of stiffness:

$$C = \frac{dV}{dp} \qquad (8.1.3)$$

$$Compliance = \frac{1}{dp / dV} = \frac{1}{stiffness} \qquad (8.1.4)$$

Thus, a more compliant the pressure transducer means that volume displacement (dV) of its diaphragm is greater when subjecting to the same amount of applied pressure (dp). The consequence of this in the accuracy of blood pressure recording is explained below. The compliance of the needle (typically made of stainless steel with high Young's modulus of elasticity and therefore, very stiff) is negligible. Equation (8.1.1) can be re-written as:

$$f_n = \frac{1}{2\pi} \sqrt{\frac{1}{LC}} \qquad (8.1.5)$$

When the needle is narrow, the Poiseuille resistance, R, becomes important in the determination of the frequency response. A second-order RLC system representation is necessary.

As we have seen in earlier chapters that blood pressure waveform is periodic and can be represented by a Fourier series as the sum of a mean pressure and a number of sine waves of fundamental frequency f (heart rate/sec) and harmonics, nf ($n = 1,2, \ldots, N$):

$$p(t) = \overline{p} + \sum_{n=1}^{N} p_n \sin(n\omega t + \phi_n) \qquad \omega = 2\pi f \qquad (8.1.6)$$

which, when substituted into the second order differential equation describing the fluid motion, results in the amplitude ratio for the nth harmonic:

$$\frac{P_{mn}}{P_{on}} = \sqrt{\frac{1}{1 - (n\omega)^2 LC + (n\omega RC)^2}} \qquad (8.1.7)$$

its corresponding phase angle:

$$\phi_n = \tan^{-1}\frac{n\omega RC}{1 - n\omega LC} \qquad (8.1.8)$$

where P_{mn} = measured pressure for the nth harmonic and P_{on} = actual pressure of the nth harmonic component. For a distortion-free blood pressure measurement system, or one with a flat frequency response, it is necessary that the amplitude ratio P_{mn}/P_{on} =1.0, or there is no difference between the measured pressure and the actual pressure. Under this condition, the phase angle ϕ_n = 0, i.e., there is no phase shift between the two.

For the pressure measurement system to record the arterial blood pressure waveform faithfully, it must have sufficient dynamic frequency response (Li *et al.*, 1976). This often results in changing the needle size or length of the needle, especially when an additional pressure transducer of different compliance specification is unavailable.

8.1.2 *Experimental Evaluation of the Frequency Response of Catheter-Pressure Transducer Systems*

For a catheter-pressure transducer system, frequently an underdamped system, compliance as well as geometric factors are important. Figure 8.1.1 provides a lumped approximation of the system. The above second-order representation can be applied to evaluate dynamic frequency response of the system.

Either a sinusoidal pressure generator or a step-response "pop-test" are common methods to evaluate dynamic frequency response of the catheter system.. Commonly, a step increase in pressure is applied against the catheter-transducer system and the balloon which is connected to the same chamber as the catheter is inflated. The balloon is then rapidly "popped" (thus, pop-test) with a sharp needle. The pressure in the chamber thus falls to atmospheric pressure, completing the step decrease in pressure. If the catheter system had a perfect dynamic response, then its response would follow exactly the step decline in pressure. However, clinically and experimentally used catheter-transducer combinations are usually underdamped, resulting in oscillations in amplitudes.

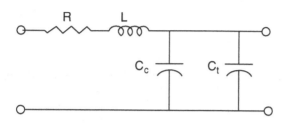

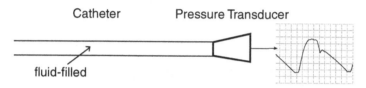

Fig. 8.1.1: Lumped model representation of the catheter-manometer system (top) and its practical recording with a fluid-filled catheter and a pressure transducer (bottom). R= Poiseuille resistance of the fluid in the catheter. C = compliance combination of the catheter and the manometer or pressure transducer (C=C_c+C_t; C_c=compliance of the catheter and C_t= compliance of the transducer). L = inertia of fluid.

The damped natural resonance frequency, f_d is obtained as the inverse of the period of oscillation:

$$f_d = \frac{1}{T} \qquad (8.1.9)$$

where T is the period of oscillation. This can be obtained from the interval of the peak-to-peak or trough-to-trough oscillations. The exponential damping, α_e is determined from the peak amplitudes A_1 and A_2,

$$\frac{A_1}{A_2} = e^{-\alpha_e t} \tag{8.1.10}$$

or in terms of amplitude ratio, A_p,

$$A_p = \ln\frac{A_2}{A_1} \tag{8.1.11}$$

The relative damping factor, α_d, is obtained from the following expression:

$$\alpha_d = \frac{A_p}{\sqrt{4\pi^2 + A_p^{\,2}}} \tag{8.1.12}$$

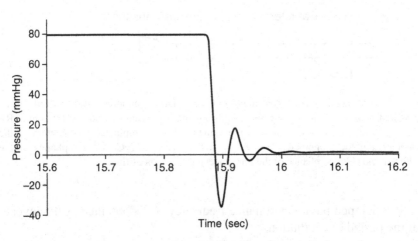

Fig. 8.1.2: The pop-test (step response) for the dynamic testing of transducer system performance, $f = 1/T$ = resonant frequency. The catheter transducer system is seen to be an underdamped system.

Most catheter-manometer systems exhibit underdamped responses, where the damping factors are low, typically of 0.1-0.3. The useful frequency range can be estimated by multiplying the resonant frequency by the damping factor. For instance, if the resonant frequency is 45 Hz and the damping factor is 0.2, then the "useful flat frequency range" is 35×0.2 or 9 Hz. The flat frequency response refers to an amplitude ratio (equation (8.1.7)) within $\pm5\%$ of unity, or 1. In other words, the measured pressure is within ±5% of the actual pressure. Thus, higher resonant frequencies and greater damping factors (up to critical damping) offer better dynamic frequency response.

The step response or pop-test has its advantages of simplicity and rapid tracking of system response. This "pop test" or step response method is shown in Fig. 8.1.2. One can apply either a positive step (step increment in pressure) or a negative step (step decrement in pressure). An ideal blood pressure measurement system would follow the step decrease in pressure exactly, with no overshoot or undershoot or time delay. In practice, however, overshoot and oscillations are common. Fig. 8.1.2 also illustrates the underdamped response of a fluid-filled catheter-manometer system. The dynamic frequency response in terms of relative amplitude ratio vs. frequency for the step response of Fig. 8.1.2 is shown in Fig. 8.1.3. The single resonance peak occurs as the underdamped catheter-manometer system was approximated by the second order system.

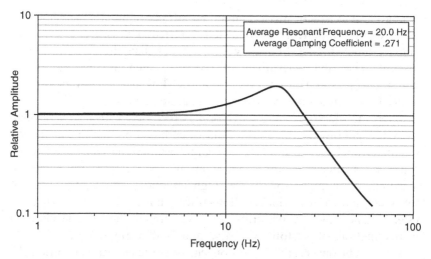

Fig. 8.1.3: Dynamic frequency response shown as the relative amplitude ratio vs. frequency. The resonance frequency in this example is 20 Hz. The damping coefficient is 0.271, indicating an underdamped blood pressure measurement system.

In general, linearity, hysteresis, and dynamic system response are necessary considerations in fluid-filled blood pressure measurement systems. Linearity refers to the output response vs. input applied pressure, obtained from static calibrations. This is not generally a problem, since most combinations have static calibrations that are linear to within ±1% or better, over the range of 0-200 mmHg. Hysteresis refers to the differences in outputs with increasing and decreasing blood pressure within the blood pressure range of interest. This is also typically small. Thus, dynamic frequency response is of the major importance.

Blood pressure waveforms that are closer to sinusoidal waveforms require less harmonic components to resynthesize the original waveform and thus place less stringent demand on the frequency response. For instance, the femoral artery can be recorded with a lower dynamic frequency response than either central aortic pressure of left ventricular pressure. This is because the femoral arterial pressure is generally smoother and with rounded dicrotic notch. Blood pressure waveforms that are closer to rectangular waveform require much higher frequency response to resynthesize the waveforms accurately. This is because rectangular and square waves contain an infinite number of sinusoidal or cosinusoidal components. Normal left ventricular pressure, for instance contains much higher frequency components than the femoral arterial pressure. The first derivatives of pressure, such as the rate of left ventricular pressure rise LV dp/dt, or aortic flow acceleration dQ/dt, also require higher frequency response for accurate recording.

When the blood pressure waveform is recorded with a low resonant frequency and low damping ratio fluid-filled blood pressure measurement system, erroneous phase shifts and large oscillations can be observed. Figure 8.1.4 illustrates this point with the aortic pressure waveform measured simultaneously by a high fidelity catheter-tip pressure transducer and a low fidelity fluid-filled catheter-pressure transducer system. The two waveforms are calibrated and superimposed. Overestimation of systolic pressure and underestimation of diastolic pressure can be observed. In addition, end-systolic pressure at aortic valve closure, systolic, diastolic and ejection periods cannot be accurately determined.

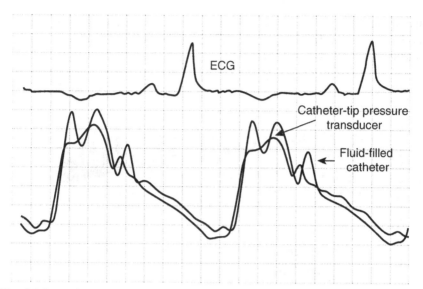

Fig. 8.1.4: Aortic blood pressure waveform measured with an underdamped catheter-manometer system and a high-fidelity catheter-tip pressure transducer. Overshoot, oscillations and associated errors in systolic pressure, diastolic pressure and timing of aortic valve closure as indicated by the dicrotic notch, are clearly seen.

Li and Noordergraaf (1977) analyzed responses of differential pressure transducer systems. For these systems, the individual frequency response, as well as static and dynamic imbalances are important factors to be considered. The efficacy of catheterization in the diagnostic setting has also been discussed by Li and Kostis (1984).

Catheter-tip pressure transducers offer superior frequency response, sufficient even for cardiac sound recording. They, however, suffer from fragility, temperature-sensitivity, and the need to be calibrated against known manometric systems. Because of their accuracy, it has replaced many of the fluid-filled catheter systems in the clinical setting.

8.2 Noninvasive Blood Pressure Measurements

8.2.1 *Auscultation Measurement of Blood Pressure*

The Korotkoff sound auscultation method remains the most popular form of noninvasive blood pressure measurement in the clinical setting. This method however, lacks accuracy when compared to invasive catheter technique. Errors of 5-10 mmHg error is common. This technique, however, is simple to employ and has surprisingly high repeatability. It allows both systolic and diastolic pressures to be determined.

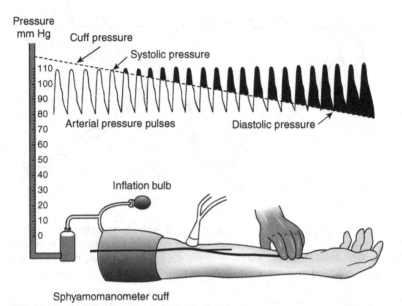

Fig. 8.2.1: Illustration of the auscultatory method for recording blood pressure. From Rushmer (1972).

Figure 8.2.1 illustrates the modern auscultation method. The cuff is inflated to a pressure exceeding the expected systolic arterial pressure (P_s). During the inflation of the cuff with cuff pressure exceeding that of the systolic pressure, the segment of the artery under the cuff is forced to collapse, either partially or completely. The cuff is then allowed to deflate slowly at a few mmHg per second. This is accomplished through a needle valve which allows air to escape, hence dropping the cuff pressure. During deflation, the initial arterial lumen opening that is is detected is the systolic pressure. The first vascular sounds that emerge is generally referred to as phase 1, define P_s. When either the vascular sounds become muffled (phase IV) or disappear completely (phase V), the diastolic pressure (P_d) is obtained. This technique has an estimated accuracy of 5-10 mmHg. There remains debate as to whether phase IV or V is a better indicator of diastolic pressure.

Figure 8.2.2 illustrates the Korotkoff vascular sounds recorded in a brachial artery. When vascular reactivity is altered with hand-grip, the spectral content is shifted, such that the Korotkoff sound intensity is increased, together with a higher observed blood pressure (Fig. 8.2.2; Matonick and Li, 1999).

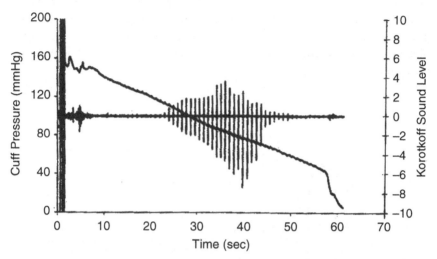

Fig. 8.2.2: Korotkoff vascular sounds recorded in a brachial artery.

The width and length of the cuff are important considerations in the application of the auscultation method, typically a width to circumference ratio of 0.4 is used. There is an optimum width of the cuff, narrower than optimum cuffs tend to impose an arterial stress below that of cuff pressure and can result in an overestimation of blood pressure. A wider cuff than optimum provide accurate recording only at the center of the cuff and can cause error in detection as stress declines away from the center, giving a lower estimation of pressure.

Numerous theories have been proposed as to the generation of the Korotkoff sounds. Their origins have been a controversial subject of research. Some have suggested that they are pressure-related rather than flow-related (Drzewiecki *et al.*, 1987).

8.2.2 Blood Pressure Measurement with the Oscillometric Method

Alternative to the use of the stethoscope is the oscillometric method. Marey in 1885 found that cuff pressure oscillated over a considerable range of mean cuff pressures. He suggested that the oscillation is maximal when the arterial wall is not stressed circumferentially. Removal of this circumferential stress, provides a basis for noninvasive tonometry. This is "vascular unloading", as Marey termed it. The tension within the wall of the artery under such circumstance is zero when the transmural pressure is zero. The maximal oscillation was found to correspond to mean arterial pressure. The oscillometric method continued to gain popularity, although this technique is rather accurate for systolic and mean blood pressure detection, its accuracy is much less so for diastolic pressure measurement.

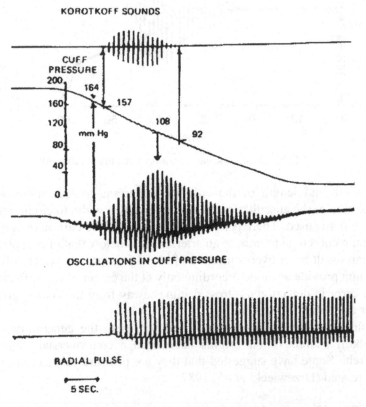

Fig. 8.2.3: Korotkoff sounds recorded concurrently with cuff pressure. Maximum oscillation in cuff pressure corresponds to mean blood pressure as shown. Radial arterial pulse distal to the brachial artery measurement site is also shown. From Geddes (1984).

Geddes (1984) has provided a detailed analysis and comparison of the cuff technique and oscillometry. Figure 8.2.3 shows the corresponding appearance and disappearance of the Korotkoff sounds and the oscillations in cuff pressure. Maximum oscillation in cuff pressure corresponds to mean blood pressure as shown. Thus, in addition to systolic and diastolic pressures, mean blood pressure can be obtained. The radial pulse distal to brachial artery measurement site is also shown.

8.2.3 *Noninvasive Blood Pressure Monitoring with Tonometer*

There are several methods for noninvasive recording of blood pressure waveforms, including the volume pulse method, the pressure pulse method, the cantilever and optical deflection methods.

In the volume pulse method (Fig. 8.2.4) successful recording hinges on the relationship between intravascular pressure distension and radial artery displacement. The pressure pulse method (Fig. 8.2.4), such as the tonometer, is dependent on the interplays of contact stress, the deformation stress and arterial pressure. Arterial pressure is actually a fraction of the contact stress. Drzewiecki *et al.* (1983) have shown that in arterial tonometery, with arterial flattening, shear stress becomes negligible compared with the normal stress in the arterial wall and skin, and uniform contact stress is developed over the transducer-skin interface. This is the ideal state for pulse recording with tonometry. Arterial tonometry for measuring blood pressure is based on the principle that when a pressurized blood vessel is partially collapsed by an external object, the circumferential stresses in the vessel wall are removed and the internal and external pressures are equal. Since tonometers are basically force transducers, they are useful only when applied to superficial arteries with solid bone backing.

Selection of pressure sensors for tonometry operation can often be a deciding factor governing sensitivity and accuracy. Many of these are solid-state or semiconductor based and their frequency responses typically well exceed the frequency contents of the underlying arterial pressure waveforms. They are light weight and comparatively less expensive. Positioning of the pressure sensors and subsequent signal conditioning are usually more of a challenge. Figure 8.2.5 illustrates such a high-fidelity tonometer recorded blood pressure waveforms over a radial artery in our laboratory. The periodic waveforms exhibit distinct features associated with systole and diastole.

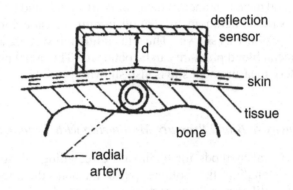

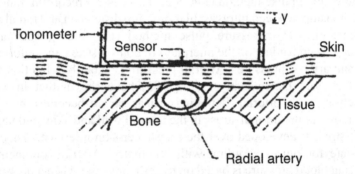

Fig. 8.2.4: Illustration of the volume pulse method (top) and the pressure pulse method (bottom). Notice the difference in the sensor placement.

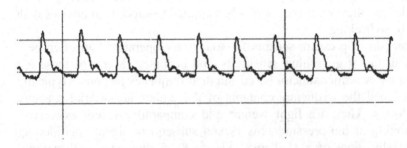

Fig. 8.2.5: Illustration of the radial artery blood pressure waveforms recorded with a high-fidelity semiconductor pressure sensor. Systolic and diastolic wave components are clearly visible.

8.2.4 *The Photoplethysmograph (PPG)*

Photoplethysmograph (PPG), is an optical measurement technique that detects pulsatile blood volume changes in the microvascular bed of the tissue. The pulsatile component is normally separated from steady components to allow the waveform to be continuously recorded for hemodynamic measurement, such as pulse transit time (PTT) or pulse wave velocity (PWV). For pulse oximeter applications, both steady (DC) and pulsatile (AC) components are required for computation of oxygen saturation. PPG employs a light emitting diode and a photo-detector which can be a photo-diode or a photo-transistor. Selection of their optical wavelength of operation is important. Typically, the emitter-detector pair is in the red wavelength range, although matched emitter-detector pairs in the near infrared (NIR) range has also been popular.

PPG is most popularly placed at the index finger, but dual PPG system placed at the superficial carotid and radial arterial sites are the most common for clinical pulse wave velocity measurements to infer vascular stiffness changes. PPG is light weight, inexpensive and easy to operate. But the recorded blood volume pulsation waveform is not an equivalent to the arterial pressure pulse. Several methods have thus been proposed to derive systolic and diastolic pressure information from the recorded PPG signals.

8.3 Blood Flow Measurement

8.3.1 *Electromagnetic Flowmeter*

In-vivo accurate measurement of blood flow lagged behind that of pressure for decades. The electromagnetic flowmeter is based on Faraday's law of induction:

$$e = v \times B - J / \sigma_c \qquad (8.3.1)$$

where the induced electric field is E, in a conductor moving with a velocity v in a magnetic field intensity *B*. *J* is the current density and σ_c is the conductivity (of blood). Figure 8.3.1 illustrates the principle. Bevir's (1971) virtual current theory, however, presents a more practical analysis.

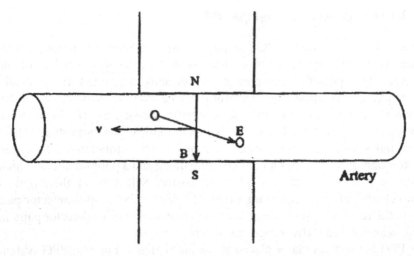

Fig. 8.3.1: Illustration of the electromagnetic blood flow measurement principles. The moving conductor (blood with velocity, v) in a magnetic field (B) induces an electric motive force and the potential (E) is picked up by the electrodes.

Wyatt (1984) reviewed blood flow and velocity measurement by electromagnetic induction. The cannula flowmeters with uniform field and point electrodes have the defect of a high degree of dependence on velocity distribution when they are not symmetric. The perivascular flowmeters have two defects: in addition to their sensitivity to velocity distribution, they are also sensitive to wall conductivity effects. The former can be reduced by using insulated- or multiple-electrodes which improve the signal-to-noise ratio. Mills' (1966) catheter-tip flowmeter has the advantage that it is unaffected by the vessel wall. Boccalon *et al.* (1978) devised a noninvasive electromagnetic flowmeter for useful clinical applications. However, the invasiveness has made the use of electromagnetic flowmeter almost obsolete in clinical situations, replaced by ultrasound Doppler.

Accurate flow measurement with an electromagnetic flow probe is by no means easy as invasive isolation of the blood vessel is required for placement of an appropriate sized flow probe to be cuffed around the vessel. Limited by available probe sizes for fitting individual blood vessels coupled with the necessity of anesthesia induced changes during the experiment, accuracy of recorded flow waveforms can be variable. The non-circular size of the pulmonary aorta and large veins make electromagnetic flow measurements even more challenging. Figure 8.3.2

demonstrates a well-recorded aortic flow in our laboratory, with minimal noise or distortion. Such phasic flow is desirable in hemodynamic studies.

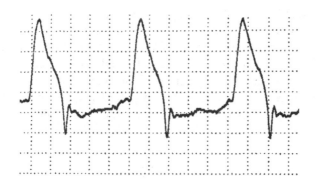

Fig. 8.3.2: Ascending aortic flow recorded with an electromagnetic flow probe. Rapid ejection to peak flow followed by reduced flow is seen. The reverse flow immediately after aortic valve closure represents flow to the coronary arteries which are perfused mostly in diastole.

8.3.2 Ultrasound and Doppler Flow Velocity Measurement

Ultrasonic methods of measuring blood flow velocity are based on either the transmission or the reflection of ultrasound. Ultrasound propagation velocity through biological tissue is about 1560 m/s. Its associated wavelength can be easily calculated from

$$\lambda = \frac{c}{f} \qquad (8.3.2)$$

Typical diagnostic ultrasound utilizes frequencies in the range of 1 MHz to 15 MHz. Thus, the corresponding wavelengths are 0.78 mm and 0.156 mm, respectively.

The transit-time ultrasound measurement of blood velocity utilizes two crystal transducers placed at two different locations, serving as transmitter and receiver. With known ultrasound velocity, c, and the transit time $\Delta t = t_1 - t_2$, we have:

$$\Delta t = \frac{2vD}{c^2 \cos \theta} \qquad (8.3.3)$$

where $D/\cos\theta$ is the distance between the transceiver and θ is the angle between the axial blood velocity and the transceiver.

A more common approach is the ultrasound Doppler technique, based on the back scattering of ultrasound by red blood cells. Turbulence, therefore, increases the scattering. Two commonly used types are continuous wave Doppler (CWD) and pulsed wave Doppler (PWD). In the CW mode, the Doppler shifted frequency, f_d, of the back scattered ultrasound is:

$$f_d = \frac{2v \cos \theta}{c} \cdot f_0 \qquad (8.3.4)$$

where v is the blood velocity, θ is the angle between the ultrasound beam and the centerline, and f_0 is the transmitted ultrasound frequency. In the PW mode, a velocity profile across the vessel can be obtained. Signal from cells scatters in a range at a depth of:

$$z = \frac{ct_d}{2} \qquad (8.3.5)$$

By pulse the ultrasound beam, one can obtain range resolution along the beam. Generally, a short burst of ultrasound is transmitted with a repetition frequency f. The backscattered signal is received and sampled after a time delay td.

Velocity profiles can also be obtained by the use of thermal-convection velocity sensors, such as hot-wire anemometers. Thermistors have been popular thermal velocity probes mounting on either a catheter or a needle. These sensors have been applied to clinical settings (Roberts, 1972).

In general, Doppler measured blood flow velocity (Fig. 8.3.3) compares well with that obtained by electromagnetic method (e.g. Yao and Pearce, 1991). Recently, high frequency ultrasound have found it place in cardiovascular diagnosis. This often requires specific array transducer design with specific materials (Shung, 2005). Hartley *et al.* (1995) developed the first Doppler velocity probe for aortic flow velocity measurement in mice and subsequently designed a high frequency (20 MHz) pulsed (125 KHz repetition rate) Doppler and catheter-based system for coronary flow reserve assessment (Hartley *et al.*, 2008). Clarity on overall cardiovascular structure (Shung, 2005) have also benefitted from ultrasound tissue characterization and strain measurements.

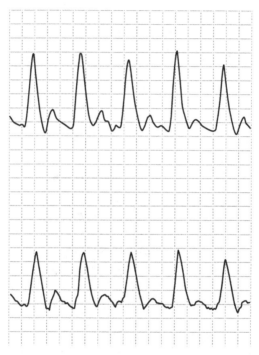

Fig. 8.3.3: Doppler ultrasound measured radial arterial blood flow velocity that is wirelessly transmitted (top) and received (bottom) with 4:3 scaling factor.

Phase contrast magnetic resonance imaging (PC-MRI) has become common for pulsatile blood flow measurement, while underlying blood vessel morphology is delineated. This involves the applications of gradient pulses that induce phase shifts in moving protons that are directly proportional to their velocity in the gradient direction. Once the peak velocity encoding value and the sensitivity and direction are specified, flow velocity can be calculated based on phase difference in the encoded images. Ascending aortic flow velocity has been obtained in this manner (Chirinos *et al.*, 2014; Phan *et al.*, 2016).

8.3.3 *Cardiac Output Measurement with Indicator Dilution Methods and Thermodilution*

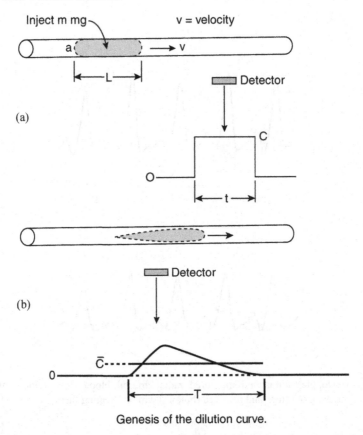

Genesis of the dilution curve.

Fig. 8.3.4: Principle of the dye dilution technique and the genesis of the dye dilution curve of concentration vs. time. From Geddes (1984).

Quantification of blood flow, even in the microcirculation by the introduction of indicators to the circulatory system has been exercised for quite some time. Dye dilution has been used for many decades. The indicator dilution method for measurement of blood flow is well illustrated in Fig. 8.1.11 (Geddes, 1984) in which an indicator of known mass is injected upstream. With the velocity of blood flow, the indicator is diluted and its concentration is detected and sampled downstream. The amount of flow, Q, is calculated from the following relation:

$$Q = \frac{m}{C_c \times t} \qquad (8.3.6)$$

where m is the mass of the injectate, C_c is the concentration, and t is time.

The Stewart-Hamilton principle states that if a known concentration of indicator is introduced into a flow stream and its temporal concentration is measured at a downstream site, then the volume flow can be calculated. The Stuart-Hamilton principle relates the flow (Q) to the mass (m) of indicator injected and the concentration (c(t)) of the indicator measured downstream at time t:

$$Q = \frac{m}{\int_0^\infty c(t)dt} \qquad (8.3.7)$$

Thus, if the area under the concentration vs. time curve is found, flow can be easily obtained. For measurement of blood flow in a single vessel, the above formulation works well. When applied to measuring cardiac output, however, the continuous pumping of the heart introduces the problem of recirculation. To overcome this, an exponential extrapolation of the concentration-time curve's descending limb is imposed such that an approximation of the integral with the area under the curve is achieved.

Indicators that have commonly been used include Evans blue dye, Indocyanine green and some radioactive isotopes, such as Albumin Iodide131. The advantage of the non-toxicity and affordability of repeated determinations within a short time span makes cold solutions excellent choices as indicators. This was demonstrated by Fronek and Ganz (1960) in the measurement of flow in single vessels including cardiac output by local thermodilution. The advent of thermodilution has made cold saline and dextrose popular indicators.

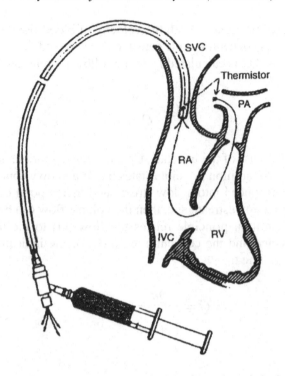

Fig. 8.3.5: Thermodilution method in man. The injection catheter is in the superior vena cava (SVC). The thermistor for measurement of indicator temperature is inside the injection catheter 1 to 2 cm from the tip. The thermistor for measurement of blood temperature is in a main branch of the pulmonary artery (PA). RA and RV are right atrium and right ventricle, respectively.

In thermodilution normal saline or isotonic dextrose (5%) in water is used as the injectate, either at 0°C or at room temperature. The most popular site of injection is the right atrium and the sampling site is the pulmonary artery. By this choice of the sites, the effect of recirculation is minimized. In this approach, a flow-directed balloon-tipped catheter can be introduced into a vein and upon inflation of the balloon, the catheter is guided with the flow into the right atrium, the right ventricle or the pulmonary artery. The thermodilution catheter typically has a thermistor near the tip of the catheter to monitor sampling site temperature. The faster the flow, the greater the temperature increase.

Ganz *et al.* (1971) demonstrated this method (Fig. 8.3.5) by injecting a 10 ml of cold (0.5-5°C) isotonic dextrose solution into the superior vena cava of a patient with normal circulation. The injectate was delivered in 1-2 seconds. The area under the thermal curve was found by planimetry which is now substituted with an analog integrator or with a digital computer.

For the thermodilution technique (Li, 2000), the standard cardiac output (CO) determination in-vivo is normally calculated from the following formula:

$$CO = \frac{V_i(T_b - T_i)S_i C_i 60}{S_b C_b \int \Delta T_b(t)dt} F_c$$

(8.3.8)

where
V_i = volume of the injectate in ml
T_b, T_i = temperature of the blood and injectate, respectively
S_b, S_i = specific gravity of the blood and injectate, respectively
C_b, C_i = specific heat of blood and injectate, respectively

The ratio of $(S_i C_i)/(S_b C_b)$ is 1.08 when 5% dextrose in water is used as an indicator. This ratio is 1.10 when normal saline is used.

The indicator heat loss along the catheter between the site of injection and the delivery site is accounted for by a correction factor, F_c:

$$F_c = \frac{T_b - T_{id}}{T_b - T_i}$$

(8.3.9)

where T_{id} is the temperature of the injectate through the catheter at the delivery site. F_c has been reported to be between 0.8 and 0.9.

8.4 Measurement of Vascular Dimensions

Measurements of geometric dimensions of blood vessels, such as length, diameter and wall thickness, are of considerable importance in quantifying dynamic behavior. Strain gages are popular for length measurements. Mercury-in-silastic rubber, constantan, silicon, and germanium transducers are examples. They are based either on dimensional change or resistivity change. Change in resistance (ΔR) is derived from:

$$R = \frac{\rho_r l}{A}$$

(8.4.1)

where A is the cross-sectional area and l is the length of the strain gage wire. The fractional change in resistance is given by:

$$\frac{\Delta R}{R} = (1 + 2\sigma)\frac{\Delta l}{l} + \frac{\Delta \rho_r}{\rho_r}$$ (8.4.2)

where σ is the Poisson ratio (ratio of radial strain to longitudinal strain). The first term on the right-hand side is due to dimensional effect, the second term to piezoresistive effect. Strain gage transducers can be applied to measure length as well as pressure. In both cases, the resultant change in resistance is detected by a Wheatstone bridge circuitry. Superior resolution with high gage factors can be obtained with semiconductors.

High resolution dimension measurement can also be obtained with ultrasonic dimension gages. The disadvantage is more complex circuitry. The method requires a pair of piezoelectric transducers (1-15 MHz) either sutured or glued on to the opposite sides of a vessel for pulsatile diameter measurement or for wall thickness measurement. It is operated in the PW mode at f =I KHz. Figure 4.1.1 gave an example of dimensional measurement (cardiac muscle segment length) with the ultrasonic dimension gages. The small size of piezoelectric crystal ultrasonic dimension transducers allows their implantation for chronic and conscious animal studies. Dynamic measurements of large vessel diameter and wall thickness can be simultaneously recorded with ultrasound operating in M-mode. However, its limitation lies in boundary identification and resolution. Similar problem is encountered with angiographic recording. Magnetic resonance imaging affords high resolution, but the disadvantage of the inability to provide real time recording. Sophisticated segmentation algorithms have been developed for obtaining high resolution diagnostically useful images of structures. Recent advance in intravascular ultrasound (IVUS) provides structural detail, as well as dimension measurements.

Chapter 9

Interaction of the Heart and the Arterial System

9.1 Ventricular Outflow and the Aorta

9.1.1 *Ventricular Ejection*

Cardiac contraction which results in ventricular ejection of blood flow into the aorta occurs in systole. This corresponds to the ejection period during which the aortic valve is open (Fig. 9.1.1). This is preceded by an isovolumic contraction period when the cardiac muscles develop force and generate pressure, while the ventricular volume stays constant (hence isovolumic). Only when the ventricular pressure exceeds the aortic pressure, the aortic valve opens and ejection begins. Thus, the interaction of the left ventricle and its receiving arterial system has been argued to begin during the ejection phase. However, numerous indices of cardiac contractility to assess the strength of ventricular contraction have been proposed during the isovolumic phase, prior to ejection before aortic valve opening. The argument is that indices derived during this cardiac contraction phase are not influenced by changes in the arterial system. Some of these indices are: maximum isovolumic ventricular pressure (LVP_{isomax}) and the maximum rate of rise of left ventricular pressure, or $LVdP/dt_{max}$.

Ventricular outflow is a function of the rate of change of ventricular volume, i.e.

$$Q = \frac{dV}{dt} \qquad (9.1.1)$$

229

The ascending aorta is the principal receiving conduit and thus its properties play a dominating role in ventricular ejection. Ventricular outflow is pulsatile, due to the contractile apparatus of the ventricle. This pulsatility is preserved due to the distensibility of the aorta and its branching arteries. This pulsatility also implies that there is an oscillatory or pulsatile contribution to the vascular load of the heart.

Components of this load, as discussed in earlier chapters, are the resistance (R), compliance (C) and inertance (L) associated with blood flow and vessel wall properties. It is recognized that the aorta contributes largely to the overall arterial system compliance. The greater mass of blood ejected during systole, contributes to inertia, hence greater overall inertance. To facilitate ventricular ejection, the aorta presents the least amount of resistance. Thus, the aorta is principally responsible for overall arterial system compliance and inertance, but less so for total peripheral resistance.

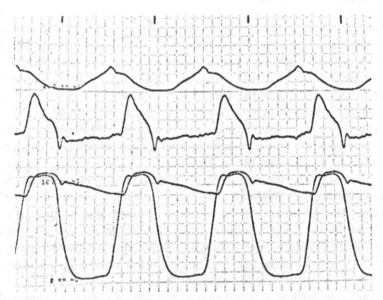

Fig. 9.1.1: Simultaneously measured cardiac muscle segment length (top tracing), aortic flow (Q), left ventricular pressure (LVP) and aortic pressure (AoP). Ejection begins when LVP exceeds AoP and ends with aortic valve closure. Cardiac muscle shortening after isovolumic ejection period to the end-systole is clearly seen.

It is important to know about the function of the heart as an energetic mechanical pump. To this end, it suffices to understand the global pressure-volume behavior in relation to cardiac muscle shortening and force generation. We shall first look at factors that give rise to ventricular ejection and then examine the factors that can modify this ejection by the aorta and the rest of the arterial system. To accomplish these, we begin with the dynamics of cardiac muscle contraction to overall ventricular pumping mechanism, and the timing and duration of the ejection. We will then look at the corresponding dynamic changes that take place in the aorta and how these changes can significantly modify ventricular outflow. As a general definition, afterload can be considered as the forces that resist ejection of the ventricular outflow. The dynamics of the vascular system thus plays a vital role in determining this outflow.

Both the left and right ventricles must eject the same amount of blood and operate synchronously. The aortic flow begins when the aortic valve is open and ends when the valve is shut. This is clearly seen in Fig. 9.1.1. Ejection is accompanied by active cardiac muscle shortening and reduced ventricular volume until end of systole.

Segmental muscle length was measured with a pair of piezoelectric ultrasound dimension gages or sonomicrometers. These gages were implanted in the myocardium about 1 cm apart with transmitting and receiving lenses facing each other. Continuous cardiac muscle segment length information is obtained by repetitive emitting and detecting the ultrasound echo time delay, hence distance, since ultrasound velocity in muscle is known.

The backflow in diastole reflects the flow to the coronary arteries perfuse the heart, mostly in diastole. Left ventricular pressure, or LVP, declines exponentially during the relaxation phase. The extent of this decline can extend to the filling phase, as during incomplete relaxation observed in coronary arterial disease. This delay can be quantified through calculation of the ventricular pressure relaxation time constant.

During the diastolic filling phase, the cardiac muscle naturally lengthens and chamber volumes increase. Diastolic filling pressure, frequently referred to as the "preload" is often used to assess the adequacy of filling. Right atrial pressure or left atrial pressure has been widely and correctly used. However, for the ease of assessing the preload, left ventricular diastolic pressure or LVEDP, is more commonly used in clinical diagnosis. Abnormally elevated LVEDP is seen in heart failure cases. As a general guideline, normal LVEDP should be lower than 12 mmHg. Significantly increased LVEDP above this value impedes the filling process and results in poorer ventricular ejection.

9.2 Cardiac Muscle Mechanics and the Force-Velocity-Length Relation

9.2.1 *Structure of Myocardial Fibers and the Sliding Filament Theory*

Sarcomeres are the fundamental building blocks of the myocardium. They exhibit the ability to change length, generate force and govern overall ventricular contraction. Within the sarcomere, there are thick and thin filaments. These are the actin and myosin molecules. The overlapping and relative positions of these filaments determine the changes in force development.

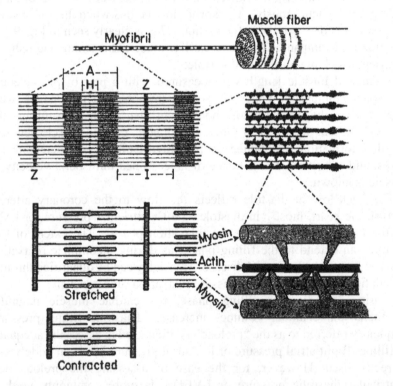

Fig. 9.2.1: Illustration of the role of the sliding filament hypothesis. The thick myosin filament and the thin actin filament are clearly seen. The overlap of actin and myosin gives rise to contraction. A-band, H-zone and Z-line are shown. From Rushmer (1972).

The "sliding filament hypothesis" as it is first proposed, formed the original basis for the understanding of the contraction process in striated muscle. This has been borrowed for cardiac muscle studies. The difference is the inherent fatigue properties observed in skeletal muscles. The tension initially increases with increasing length of the fiber, until the sarcomere reaches a length of about 2.2 μm, the tension reaches a maximum and then declines as the length is increased further. The extent of the overlapping filaments determines the amount of force generation. This scheme is illustrated in Fig. 9.2.1 (see also Sugi and Pollack, 1993).

The sarcomere tension-length relationship has been translated to the intact global heart in terms of left ventricular developed pressure (LVP) and end-diastolic volume (EDV). The former is related to the developed tension or force, while the latter is related to the initial muscle fiber length (l_0) or "preload".

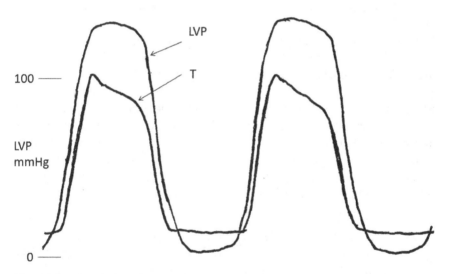

Fig. 9.2.2: Simultaneously measured regional tension (force) and global ventricular pressure in the left ventricle. Notice the parallel relationship between pressure (LVP) and tension (T) in the isovolumic phases. They differ significantly in other parts of the cardiac cycle.

The relation between sarcomere length (l) and left ventricular volume (V) however, is not a linear one. This is expected, as the left ventricle is non-cubical in shape. Thus, the percentage change in cardiac muscle fiber length cannot be interpreted as a corresponding percentage in left ventricular cavity volume. Even in the isovolumic ejection phase, when the ventricular volume remains constant, cardiac muscle fibers at different part of the ventricle may still be changing their lengths. Thus, isovolumic (constant volume) contraction does not exactly correspond to isometric (constant length) contraction. The regional tension and global ventricular pressure relationship is seen to be parallel however, only during the isovolumic contraction and relaxation phases (Fig. 9.2.2 and Li, 1987). Thus, ventricular pressure cannot be used to infer force of generation for the entire systole. It is also clear that ventricular pressure declines after tension declines from its peak.

The anisotropic properties and differential epicardial and endocardial segmental contraction due to their fiber orientations complicate the direct translation of mechanics from the muscle level to the global ventricular level. This aspect is particularly relevant in current magnetic resonance imaging studies in the quantification of regional strains (Liao *et al.*, 2003) to assess regional muscle shortening and global cardiac function.

9.2.2 Hill Model of Muscle Contraction

Much of the biomechanics of muscle contraction can be traced back to Hill, who was concerned about the mechanical efficiency, in terms of work and speed, of human muscles. Although the concept of mechanical spring as an energy storage element was introduced to model muscle behavior before him, Hill accounted for the energy dissipation through the introduction of a viscoelastic model. This leads to the expression:

$$k(l - l_0) - \beta_o \frac{dl}{dt} = F$$

$$(9.2.1)$$

where k and β_o are constants, l and l_0 are the instantaneous and the initial muscle lengths, respectively. F is the applied force. The velocity of shortening is represented by the rate of change of fiber length

$$v = \frac{dl}{dt}$$

(9.2.2)

This velocity term thus gives rise to the viscous effect. At any given muscle length l, a larger load F is lifted with a lower velocity than a smaller load. Or that the muscle can contract at a faster rate if subjected to a smaller load than a larger load. Thus, the ability to generate force and the extent of velocity of shortening of the contractile element has an inverse relationship.

Hill's two element model, consisting of a passive series elastic element and a contractile element has become popular and follows the general expression:

$$(F+a)(v+b) = k_o$$

(9.2.3)

where k_o is a constant. The velocity of shortening is a function of initial length of the muscle fiber. Combined with the earlier force-length relation, the force-velocity-length (f-v-l) relation has been suggested to be able to completely describe the physical behavior of the muscle.

9.3 The Pressure-Volume Curve and Contractility of the Heart

9.3.1 *Variables Defining the Pressure-Volume Loop*

The pressure-volume relation has been popular because it provides the inter-relationships between stroke volume (SV), end-diastolic volume (EDV), end-systolic volume (ESV) and ejection fraction (EF) on a single diagram. The pressure-volume diagram (Fig. 9.3.1) is constructed from the instantaneous recordings of left ventricular pressure and volume. In addition, it has been suggested that the separation of cardiac mechanical pump function and contractile state can be obtained. Pump function is related to loading conditions whereas contractility or inotropic state depends only on the intrinsic properties of the contracting muscle fibers or the myocardium.

The importance of P-V loop or pressure-diameter (P-D) loops of the ventricle has been frequently emphasized. This diagram points to the

ESV as one of the functional determinants of this representation of ventricular pump function. Preload is indicated by the EDV and

$$SV = EDV - ESV \qquad (9.3.1)$$

is the stroke volume. It is clear that the pressure-volume relationship provides a gross assessment of the global mechanical performance of the heart. Here, the regional volume and shape changes are not taken into account. Regional or local geometric variations are often observed through contour mapping or regional strain calculations during imaging (e.g. Liao et al., 2003).

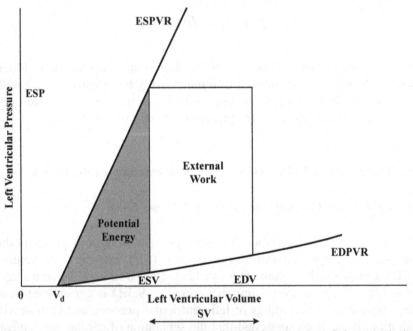

Fig. 9.3.1: Pressure-volume (P-V) diagram of the left ventricle defining ventricular elastance and V_d. The end-systolic pressure-volume line is drawn as tangent to the P-V loop at end-systole. Its slope represents the maximum elastance of the left ventricle, or E_{max}.

Another important aspect of the pressure-volume curve is the area under the loop which represents the mechanical work performed by the ventricle to overcome its vascular load. For this reason, it is often termed the external work (EW) of the heart and the area under the P-V loop is also known as the "work loop". This work loop area is approximately the product of mean aortic pressure and the stroke volume, viz.

$$EW \approx \bar{p} \times SV$$

(9.3.2)

For a normal human heart with aortic pressure of 120/80 mmHg and stroke volume of 75 ml, the external work, or stroke work, generated is about 1 Joule (10^7 ergs) per heartbeat (Li, 1986, 1996). The amount of stroke work performed by the left ventricle thus varies with blood pressure, as well as stroke volume. In chronic hypertension, for instance, stroke work can be significantly higher. In other words, the heart works harder in an attempt to maintain its stroke volume. Pressure work is more costly in terms of myocardial oxygen consumption (Li, 1982) can be seen in clinical cases of hypertension, hypertrophy and aortic stenosis, for instances. In these, the pressure-volume loops or the work-loops are much larger.

9.3.2 Frank-Starling Mechanism and Ejection Fraction

The Frank-Starling mechanism dictates that force generation, associated with a better-filled heart with a larger end-diastolic volume (EDV), results in a larger SV. Thus, ejection fraction (EF), which is the ratio of SV to EDV, represents the LV input-output relationship and subsequently places EF as a critical factor in governing overall cardiac function.

The Frank-Starling mechanism, also better known as the "Starling's Law of the Heart", has classically been regarded as a fundamental property of the ventricle to regulate its cardiac output. The larger the volume before the onset of contraction, the higher is its output under otherwise identical conditions. In this context, the preload has been identified as the filling pressure or end-diastolic volume. Figure 9.3.2 illustrates the working paradigm of the Starling's Law: as end-diastolic volume EDV, increases or with better filling, the stroke volume or SV increases. Starling's law can be expressed in terms of the ratio of the volume that is ejected to the total resting volume. This ejection fraction is defined as:

$$EF = SV / EDV \qquad (9.3.3)$$

The normal mammalian heart has an ejection fraction of 0.5 to 0.7. Table 9.3.1 provides some of the reported values of ejection fraction in different species of mammals.

Table 9.3.1: Ejection fractions in some mammalian species

Man	0.67
Dog	0.65
Cat	0.64
Rabbit	0.61

Together with cardiac output, the product of stroke volume and heart rate,

$$CO = SV \times HR \qquad (9.3.4)$$

ejection fraction has been widely used in the clinical setting as an index of LV performance.

Concerning ventricular volume regulation, Kerkhof *et al.* (2002) have further emphasized the importance of end-systolic volume in governing overall cardiac performance. "Alternative Starling's Curve", or ASC, as it is termed examined the relation between ESV and EDV, rather than SV and EDV, was obtained as a linear relationship with a much better regression:

$$ESV(I) = \alpha + \beta\, EDV(I) \qquad (9.3.5)$$

Here α and β are empirically determined constants and (I) indicates index normalized to body surface area (m^2). ESV-EDV relation takes into account of cardiac contractility as a dominant factor rather than the SV-EDV or input-output relation given by the classic Starling's Law.

Volume regulation in general has been also seen to be critical in heart failure conditions (Kerkhof *et al.*, 2013).

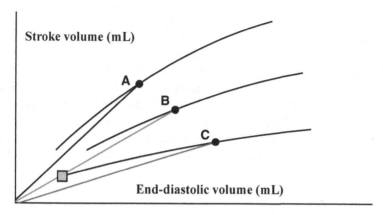

Fig. 9.3.2: Schematic examples of Starling curves. Ejection Fraction (EF) can be assessed from the curve by taking the slope of the line connecting the origin with the actual operating point (A, B, or C in this example, referring to curves with high, normal, and low contractility, respectively). Note that EF always decreases when end-diastolic volume (EDV) rises.

9.3.3 *Cardiac Contractility and Indices of Cardiac Performance*

The amount of blood ejected out of the ventricle per beat or the stroke volume is dependent not only on the operating Starling mechanism, or the preload, it is also dependent on the afterload, contractility and heart rate. We shall take a look of factors that govern cardiac contractility and indices that are used to assess cardiac performance.

Ejection fraction (EF) has long been hailed as a simple index of cardiac performance. It is a simple, dimensionless number and based upon Starling's law of the heart. Experimental studies, with volume loading or increased end-diastolic volume or filling pressure, have shown that utilization of Starling's law to be effective in improving LV function in the short term. However, when the intrinsic contractile properties change, Starling's law alone cannot explain the underlying abnormal cardiac performance. Thus, numerous indices of cardiac contractility have been proposed.

At the global level, pressure, volume and geometry are parameters which are commonly measured through catheterization and imaging. For the ease of assessing ventricular function during catheterization, each patient's electrocardiogram (ECG), cine-angiogram, LVP, and thermodilution cardiac output are normally measured. Thus, together with LVEDP, the maximum rate of rise of left ventricular pressure (LVdP/dt$_{max}$) is recorded. This latter has been routinely referred to as an "index of LV contractility" in the clinical setting. However, it has been found to be dependent on arterial system load, signifying the close coupling of the LV to the AS. To justify its use, it has been linked to the "impulse response" of the LV in terms of its outflow. Thus, this initial impulse of the ejection flow has also been used as an index of contractility. Since LVP pressure is normally measured, LVdP/dt$_{max}$ has been correlated with the maximum aortic flow (Q) acceleration or dQ/dt$_{max}$ (see Fig. 3.3.4). Unfortunately, both dP/dt$_{max}$ and dQ/dt$_{max}$ have been found to be dependent also on afterload. For instances, a decreased arterial compliance or increased peripheral resistance can change LV dP/dt$_{max}$. Their exclusive use as indices of cardiac contractility thus has met with limitations.

Alternatively, the velocity of cardiac muscle shortening has been used to describe contractility using the force-velocity-length relationship (see 9.2.2 above). This stems from Hill's original analysis of muscle contraction. For all practical purposes, the circumferential velocity of shortening, based upon an assumed elliptical geometry of the heart, has been most commonly used. Since LVP is frequently measured, this index of contractility can be defined as the maximum velocity of shortening of the contractile element or v$_{ce}$:

$$v_{ce} = \left[\frac{1}{\alpha P}\right] dP/dt \qquad (9.3.6)$$

where α is somewhat similar to a spring constant and has a value of approximately 32 cm^{-1}. In this representation, the cardiac muscle is modeled as a spring-dashpot combination.

Alternatively, from the pressure-volume (P-V) relationship (refer to Fig. 9.3.1), the end-systolic pressure-volume relation (ESPVR) is utilized to determine maximum elastance of the left ventricle, or Emax, since the slope (or elastance) defined by LV pressure and volume is maximum at end-systole:

$$Emax = ESP/(ESV - Vo) \qquad (9.3.7)$$

ESP and ESV are end-systolic pressure and volume, respectively. Vo is the residual volume, or the dead volume at which the ventricle cannot generate pressure. Since Vo can only be determined when LVP = 0, this imposes an impractical measurement in clinical situations. Thus, Vo is assumed to be 0 in many instances. Vo has been shown to vary greatly in heart failure. In addition, increased contractility is related to a reduced Vo.

Similar to the use of LVdP/dt$_{max}$, Emax has also been used extensively to reflect the contractile state of the heart. It has also been utilized in many heart failure studies. Emax has been shown to be also arterial load dependent, i.e. ESPVR becomes curvilinear at higher arterial pressures, thus making it afterload dependent. This has a consequential effect on the interaction between the LV and the arterial system, as we shall see in a later section. Emax is derived from the time-varying compliance concept in which the heart is characterized as a muscular pump. Thus, the pressure-volume relationship dictates the extent of systolic ejection. Indeed, the ejection process is dependent not only on the contractility of the LV, but also on the arterial system load it faces.

9.4 Heart and the Arterial System Interaction

9.4.1 *The Concept of Ventricular and Arterial Elastances*

In assessing the coupling and the interaction of the heart and the arterial system several methods have been proposed. To simplify the analysis, approaches have mostly been based on models with lumped parameters. One such method the arterial system is represented by an effective arterial elastance (E_a), although E_a does not directly reflect the physical elastic properties of the arteries. Elastance defined here, reflects only a system property, i.e. it does not equal the elastic properties of arteries. It is derived from the three-element Windkessel model and based on the assumption that the arterial system behaves linearly. As such, it is a steady-state parameter that incorporates peripheral resistance, arterial compliance and characteristic impedance of the aorta, and systolic and diastolic intervals,

$$E_a = \frac{R_s}{[t_s + \tau(1 - e^{-t_d/\tau})]}$$

(9.4.1)

where t_s and t_d are systolic and diastolic periods, respectively. The diastolic pressure decay time constant is shown as before,

$$\tau = R_s C$$

(9.4.2)

E_a has been approximated by the ratio of end-systolic pressure to stroke volume (SV or V_s), or

$$E_a \approx P_{es}/SV$$

(9.4.3)

When the mean arterial pressure is used to approximate P_{es}, then E_a can be easily estimated from

$$E_a = \overline{P}/V_s$$

(9.4.4)

Approximation of mean pressure to P_{es} is good under normal physiological conditions, but poor during strong vasoactive conditions.

Cardiac output is the product of stroke volume and heart rate, as

$$CO = V_z \cdot f_h$$

(9.4.5)

where

$$f_h = \frac{1}{T}$$

(9.4.6)

T is cardiac period. The effective arterial elastance can be rewritten as

$$E_a \approx \frac{R_s}{T}$$

(9.4.7)

since R_s is simply the ratio of mean arterial pressure divided by cardiac output. Alternatively, when the diastolic aortic pressure decay time constant is long compared with the diastolic period, or $\tau \gg t_d$, the denominator of equation (9.4.1) reduces to

$$t_s - \tau\,(1\text{-}1\text{-}t_d/\tau) = t_s + t_d = T \qquad (9.4.8)$$

where Taylor expansion is applied to the exponential term. When the assumption that the peripheral resistance is much larger than the characteristic impedance of the aorta, or $R_s \gg Z_o$, is also made, then the effective arterial elastance becomes, again,

$$E_a \approx \frac{R_s}{T}$$

$$(9.4.9)$$

The effective arterial system elastance obtained in this manner is only dependent on the peripheral resistance and the cardiac period. It is totally independent of the elastic properties of the arterial system.

In terms of ventricular function, a popular index used to describe its contractility is the maximal elastance (E_{max}) of the ventricle. It is derived from the ventricular pressure-volume relation (Suga *et al.*, 1973). In this context, the ventricle is modeled with a time-varying compliance, $C_v(t)$, the inverse of which is the time-varying elastance, $E(t)$. The concept of using E_{max} as an "index of cardiac contractility" is more clearly demonstrated when interventions that alter pumping ability of the heart are imposed. For instance, with epinephrine infusion, the slope increased and hence an increase in contractility.

Figure 9.4.1 gives a schematic drawing of left ventricular pressure plotted against left ventricular volume. The pressure-volume loop, or P-V loop, follows an anti-clockwise direction. It can be seen that the end-systolic points of the P-V loops lie on a straight line. This line intercepts the volume axis at Vd. At end-systole, the elastance ($E(t)$) slope is at its maximum and this defines Emax:

$$Emax = Pes/(Ves\text{-}Vo) \qquad (9.4.10)$$

where Emax is the maximum elastance of the ventricle, Ves is the end-systolic volume and Vo is the dead volume, or the volume at which the ventricle no longer has the ability to develop pressure. Neglect Vo results in a simplified relation

$$Ees = Pes / Ves \qquad (9.4.11)$$

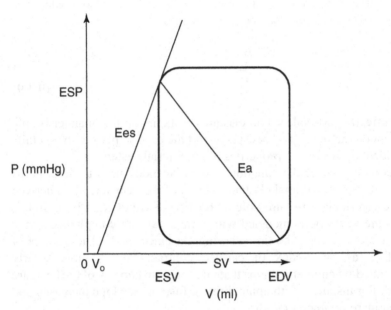

Fig. 9.4.1: Diagram defining the effective arterial elastance E_a, showing its relation to the left ventricular elastance, E_{es}. ESP is the end-systolic pressure, ESV and EDV are end-systolic and end-diastolic volumes, respectively. SV=EDV-ESV. Vo is the dead volume.

Despite its obvious limitations, the simple ratio of Ea/Ees has been used extensively to characterize the interaction of the heart and the arterial system (e.g. Kelly *et al.*, 1992; Starling, 1993). Fig. 9.4.1 illustrates the steady state coupling of the ventricle and the arterial system using the ratio of Ea/Ees (Sunagawa *et al.*, 1983).

It has been shown by that the use of peripheral vasoactive agents such as the potent vasoconstrictor methoxamine (MTX) and potent vasodilator nitroprusside (NTP), as we have shown in Chapter 4, arterial system load can be significantly increased or decreased, respectively. As a result, the ratio of E_a/E_{es} is altered, indicates changes in ventricle-arterial system coupling. With dobutamine, on the other hand, E_a stays unaltered, while E_a is increased with vasoconstrictor methoxamine and decreased with vasodilator nitroprusside (Li and Zhu, 1994). These vasoactive agents do not seem to alter the slope of the end-systolic pressure-volume line, or E_{es} (Starling, 1993; Fig. 9.4.2). Thus, the coupling ratio E_a/E_{es} can be altered by either a change in cardiac contractility or a change in arterial load.

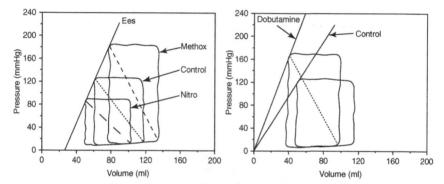

Fig. 9.4.2: Pressure-volume diagrams of the ventricle illustrating the steady state coupling of the ventricle and the arterial system using the ratio of E_a/E_{es}. With methoxamine and nitroprusside infusions, the slope of Ees is unchanged, while E_a is altered. With dobutamine infusion, Ees is increased, while E_a is unchanged. From Starling (1993).

Another aspect is related to the dynamic changes involving pulse wave velocity and wave reflections. Increases in PWV and reflection induced by MTX increased late systolic LV loading relative to control. NTP had opposite effects, i.e. unloading. Model-based experiments revealed that both increased PWV and reflections independently contribute to late systolic loading (Phan *et al.*, 2015). When PWV and reflections are both elevated, higher degree of late systolic loading. Drug therapy can have complex effects and differential efficacy in the course of treatment of hypertension. Hypertension therapy (MacFadyen, 2008) and its impact on the underlying hemodynamics is an important aspect that remains somewhat unresolved.

The effects of alterations of windkessel model parameters on the ventricular pressure-volume relation under steady state conditions have been investigated (Maughan *et al.*, 1984). The changes in arterial compliance and peripheral resistance have little effects on the slope of the end-systolic pressure-volume relation. However, the shape and the trajectory of left ventricular elastance are significantly altered, indicating temporal influences of arterial system load on LV performance.

It should be noted here that there are other indices to cardiac performance, such as the pump function curve proposed by Van den Horn *et al.* (1984), the maximum velocity of cardiac muscle shortening concept suggested by Brutsaert (1974) based on force-velocity-length relations, as shown in section 9.3.3.

9.4.2 *Dynamic Heart-Arterial System Interaction*

Blood pressure varies during the cardiac cycle. Thus, vascular compliance is also expected to vary continuously. This dynamic time-varying, pressure-dependent compliance property is incorporated in a nonlinear model of the systemic arterial system (see Section 4.5).

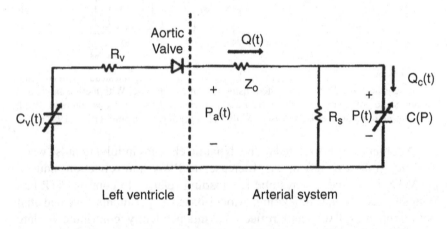

Fig. 9.4.3: Nonlinear model of the arterial system coupled to the left ventricle. $C_v(t)$ =time-varying left ventricular compliance, R_v =systolic ventricular resistance, Z_0 = aortic characteristic impedance, R_s =peripheral resistance, C(P) =pressure-dependent or dynamic arterial compliance. $P_a(t)$ and Q(t) are aortic pressure and flow, respectively. Illustration provided by Dr. Janet Ying Zhu.

A model incorporating this property to investigate the dynamic heart-arterial system interaction is shown in Fig. 9.4.3. The left ventricle is represented by a time-varying compliance and a systolic resistance. The time-varying compliance is the inverse of time-varying elastance. Both time-varying compliance of the left ventricle and the pressure-dependent compliance of the arterial system exhibit temporal dependence, hence they are dynamic in nature.

This model predicted changes have particular implications in terms of global heart-arterial system interaction. For instance, the pressure-dependent arterial compliance (C(P)) increases during the early systole to facilitate ventricular ejection, but reaches a minimum at about end-systole (Fig. 9.4.4). The dynamic elastance of the arterial system represented as the inverse of the pressure-dependent arterial system compliance is:

$$E_{as}(t) = 1/C(P)$$

$$(9.4.12)$$

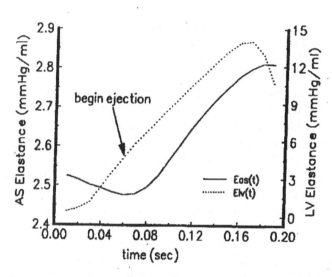

Fig. 9.4.4: Temporal relation of time-varying left ventricular and arterial system elastances, demonstrating the dynamic interaction during systole. Arterial system elastance is obtained from the pressure-dependent compliance ($E_{as}(t) = 1/C(P)$).

At end-systole, this is when both time-varying arterial elastance and ventricular elastance are at their respective maximum (Emax , also Berger and Li, 1992). The developing arterial elastance at systole reflects the time-varying compliance characteristics that are associated with active tension development of the arterial wall, as established for the ventricular muscle. This also demonstrates that the interaction of the heart and the arterial system is a dynamic one, particularly in systole. The arterial compliance thus bears a temporal, hence dynamic, relation to left ventricular function.

9.4.3 *Left Ventricle-Arterial System Interaction in Heart Failure*

In heart failure, the weakened contractile apparatus of the heart during ejection still has to face a varying afterload. This latter can be decreased large vessel compliance, an increased vascular stiffness or an increased peripheral resistance, or both. It can either compensate by increasing chamber size, via the Frank-Starling mechanism in the short term, or developing cardiac hypertrophy capable to accommodate the SV demand in the long term. Some heart failure patients, although suffering from compromised cardiac function, have frequently been observed to have their ejection fraction (EF) somewhat preserved (HFpEF). However, others have persistent reduced ejection fraction (HFrEF). Since LV ejection is dependent on the manner with which it is coupled to the arterial system, analyzing parameters governing the interaction of the LV and the AS in heart failure can be crucial in successful management of the therapeutic outcome (Kerkhof *et al.*, 2013; Li and Atlas, 2015).

About half of all patients with heart failure are diagnosed as having an almost normal EF (EF >50%) with an EDV <97 mL/m^2. This subgroup is denoted as the syndrome of heart failure with preserved EF, or HFpEF. The other half exhibits a reduced EF (<50%) which is in accordance with the classical notion that HF is reflected by a significantly decreased value of EF, or HFrEF. Thus, a normal EF may be associated with a poor cardiac condition. Therefore, EF alone cannot be a unique index for describing the performance of the heart. To resolve this dilemma, it is necessary to look into the significant differences of the arterial system behavior, or the vascular loading properties, for each of these two patient groups.

The heart, whether functioning normally or in failure, is coupled to the arterial system. The arterial system thus presents a combination of both a "steady" and a "time-varying" load to the heart; even under normal conditions. In heart failure, such loading conditions can be variably large. Reduced compliance, or increased vascular stiffness, has been observed in heart failure patients with hypertension, LV hypertrophy, aortic stenosis and coronary arterial disease. Compliance is a physical property directly dependent on the elastic behavior of the aorta. Its inverse, or vascular stiffness, is linked to the mechanical properties of the arterial wall structure.

We recently showed that Ea alone is not considered useful in assessing the severity of HF in patients with either preserved or reduced EF, and certainly cannot differentiate the two groups (Kerkhof *et al.*, 2013). The surprising evaluation outcome is that arterial compliance is significantly different and appears to be a clearly differentiable factor between the HFpEF and HFrEF groups. But EF does not seem to be exclusively dependent on arterial compliance for either of the two groups. It is obvious that heart failure patients with preserved ejection fraction display an EF that can be practically independent of changes in arterial compliance. In the heart failure patients with reduced ejection fraction, EF tends to rise with an increase in arterial compliance. Thus, in the HFrEF group, therapeutic drugs which increase arterial compliance may significantly improve overall LV-AS coupling and hence overall cardiac performance.

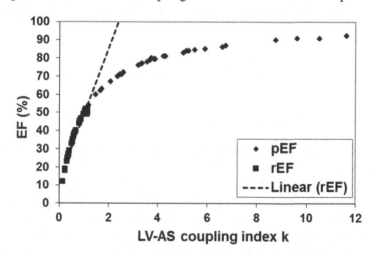

Fig. 9.4.5: Ejection fraction (EF) plotted as a function of the LV-AS coupling index (k). A linear regression line ($r^2 = 0.95$) is generally found for the HFrEF group (n=33;■). The linear line fits through the data of HFrEF group (- - -). The relationship for the HFpEF group (n=34;♦) is clearly nonlinear. Graph provided by Dr. P.L.M. Kerkhof.

Another interesting finding shows that the EF in HFrEF group of patients is highly dependent on LV-AS coupling coefficient, k (=Emax/Ea). This implies that even as EF improves in these patients, the LV-AS coupling has limited improvement (see Fig. 9.4.5). Whereas in the HFpEF patient group the LV-AS coupling can be significantly improved with just slight improvement in EF (Fig. 9.4.5).

Here we have primarily focused on the hemodynamic events associated with the LV-AS interaction in HF, we must also recognize that some of the neurohumoral mechanisms may significantly impact the vascular system and the heart. For instance, increased activity of the renin-angiotensin-aldosterone system (RAAS) in HF and other underlying pathological mechanisms, can play a dominant role in adverse vascular remodeling. In addition, over-stimulation by the sympathetic system has been a major concern in HF patients. This has led to selective beta-adrenergic receptor blockade for treatment. While beta-blockers have long been shown to be effective in treating hypertensive patients, the use of angiotensin converting enzyme inhibitors (ACE inhibitors) has also been shown to be effective (MacFadyen *et al.*, 1993). Thus, the interplay of neurohumoral mechanisms and hemodynamics may eventually determine the optimum strategy for successful treatment of heart failure patients.

9.5 Heart-Arterial System Interaction in the Assisted Circulation

9.5.1 *Mechanical Assist Devices and the Intra-Aortic Balloon Pump*

The heart is generally viewed as an energetic mechanical pump. As such, a means to assist its function under adverse conditions need to be mechanical in nature. With limited donors for heart transplants and the limited success with long term use of artificial hearts (although the most recent patient survived about 4 months), other avenues of cardiac assistance for a failing heart take center-stage. Mechanical assistance and replacements for damaged hearts have grown in application in recent years and is expected to grow in the near future. While many problems have developed during clinical studies of total artificial hearts, artificial heart assist devices appear to operate without such extensive difficulties. The versatility of such devices are in their varied designs to be either temporary or permanent, internal or external and can operate in a number of modes relative to the natural heart. The most common mode for implantable heart assist devices is to operate in parallel with the left ventricle with blood pumped from the left atrium to the ascending aorta. In this mode (parallel to the left ventricle) the assist device can take over varying percentages of the pumping work and blood flow.

Intra-aortic balloon pump or IABP is perhaps the most commonly employed temporary mechanical assist device in the clinical setting. The IABP is placed in-series with the left ventricle. Its use serves as an ideal topic for studying the heart-arterial system interaction in an assisted circulation. The IABP is surgically inserted into the descending thoracic aorta below the aortic arch and is operated in a counterpulsation mode (Fig. 9.5.1). In this type of operation the balloon is inflated to assist retrograde aortic flow into the coronary arteries during diastole when the aortic valve is closed and deflated during systole when the natural heart is pumping. Timing of the inflation and deflation of the balloon is considered the most important determinant of overall efficacy.

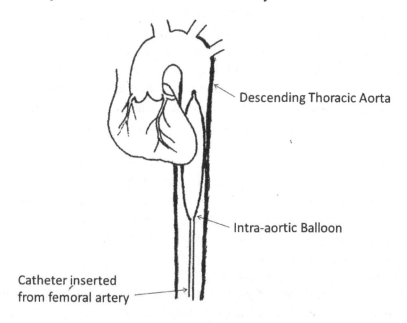

Fig. 9.5.1: illustration of the placement of intra-aortic balloon pump in the descending aorta. Inflation in diastole and deflation in systole constitutes the basis of counterpulsation in-series cardiac assistance.

Some of the bypass devices have been utilized as temporary assist devices and in-series devices have been utilized as permanent assist devices. In all of the applications, the control of the device timing relative to the natural heart is quite critical. While for temporary devices manual controls are, in many cases, acceptable, it is clear that for permanent implanted devices, automatic, and preferably implantable, controls are essential. Many of the attempts at automatic control of heart assist devices were studied in conjunction with IABP since the balloon pumps are widely used in the clinical setting.

As mentioned above, the intra-aortic balloon pump and its control reflect an excellent example of the dynamic interaction of the heart and the vascular system. The heart pumps blood into the arterial system only during systole, while diastole occupies the remaining period. Many investigators recognized that the possibility of providing additional flow to vital organ vascular beds, including the coronaries, exists during diastole. This observation enables mechanical assistance designed to improve blood flow supplied by a failing ventricle through proper timing. The intra aortic balloon pump (IABP) was introduced to modify aortic pressure in a pulsatile manner, first in dogs and later in humans in the 1960's. An elongated balloon is inserted via the superficial femoral artery and advanced to the descending aorta. Deflation in systole and inflation in diastole produces in-series assistance. A variation is a device that directs blood from the failing ventricle to the aorta, thus producing parallel assistance.

IABP has most widely been used in patients with either cardiogenic shock (Pierce *et al.*, 1981; Waksman *et al.*, 1993) after acute myocardial infarction (Mueller, 1994; Ohman *et al.*, 1994; Ishihara *et al.*, 1994) or left ventricular failure after cardiac surgery. The beneficial aspects in terms of hemodynamics are the decreased systolic afterload, augmented diastolic aortic pressure, increased cardiac output, reduced left ventricular size, and improved myocardial metabolism.

Some of the direct and immediate beneficial effects of IABP have been the reduction of epicardial segment elevation and limitation of the spread of myocardial infarct, reduced S-T segment elevation and reduced infarcted zone area. In addition, mortality and morbidity associated with acute myocardial infarction might also be decreased by IABP. However, when IABP is initiated in a delayed fashion, i.e. six hours after the onset of symptoms of transmural myocardial infarction accompanied by acute heart failure, IABP does not seem to alter myocardial infarct size, nor to alter morbidity or mortality in patients. Thus, the hemodynamic and cardiac electrophysiological beneficial effects and success rate of mechanical assistance are higher, the earlier the application of such devices.

Li *et al.* (1984) and others have examined the hemodynamic effects of IABP in terms of ultrasonic dimension gauges recorded cardiac muscle shortening. These miniature piezoelectric crystals were implanted typically in the subendocardium of the left ventricle in the normal, border, and ischemic zones. Pumping was initiated at various times after the onset of coronary artery occlusion. Contraction, assessed by segmental muscle shortening was significantly improved in the border zone, but unchanged either in the central ischemic zone, or in the normal zone. This was attributed to the border zone regional increase in myocardial blood flow and in the availability of oxygen due to augmented diastolic perfusion pressure.

There are disputes as to which appropriate hemodynamic variables are suitable as controls to optimize the efficacy of cardiac assist devices (CADs) either in-series or in-parallel. Two such variables utilized are the aortic pressure and the cardiac output. Their use as input control signals has been found to be inadequate from both experimental and model studies.

Apart from IABP, left ventricular assist devices (LVADs) exist in several types. They may be either pulsatile or non-pulsatile, synchronous or non-synchronous to the pumping of the natural heart. These may be the sac type, the diaphragm type, the pusher-plate type, the roller pump, or the centrifugal pump type.

The LVADs are used in patients with either reversible or nonreversible cardiac failure and can be used for temporary or permanent assistance. These types of cardiac assist devices are sometimes referred to as parallel assist devices or bypass devices because they direct blood from either the left atrium or the left ventricle to the aorta, hence acting in parallel with the natural heart pump. As with all cardiac assist devices, the primary aim of the LVAD is to provide adequate perfusion to vital organ vascular beds. Of secondary concern is to unload the heart, or to reduce afterload and hence myocardial oxygen consumption.

Blood pressure is often higher when the LVAD is on rather than off. This tends to increase the load on the left ventricle, which is already in failure with reduced external work capability. The counterpulsation mode allows the reduction of afterload however, if properly synchronized. Synchronous actuation, with left ventricular apical cannulation, provides the greatest amount of ventricular unloading. Nevertheless, synchronization does not appear to be a priority of many of the designs of cardiac assist devices, whose primary use are to maintain adequate cardiac output.

9.5.2 *Optimization of Intra-Aortic Balloon Pumping: Physiological Considerations*

The major hemodynamic aims and consequently the benefits of IABP are the increase in coronary perfusion and the reduction of ventricular afterload, hence an increase in cardiac efficiency. The extent of these benefits is dependent upon a number of physical and physiological parameters. These include the position of the balloon in the aorta, the volume displacement and its geometric size relative to the aorta, the driving gas, the rates and timing of balloon inflation and deflation, the heart rate, the viscoelastic properties of the aorta, neural-humoral influences, and the severity of the heart failure.

Theoretically speaking, the optimal position for the intra aortic balloon should be as close to the aortic valve as possible, in order to generate the augmentation of mean arterial diastolic pressure (P_d) to enhance coronary perfusion. But this positioning obstructs flow to the aortic arch vessels. Thus, the ideal position chosen is normally along the descending throracic aorta just distal to the arch. Balloon volume determines the absolute magnitude of changes in hemodynamic parameters. Experimental studies indicate that diastolic pressure augmentation through volume displacement also enables one to effectively lower peak ventricular pressure and myocardial oxygen consumption due to the rapid balloon collapse prior to the following ventricular systole.

The effects of balloon geometry indicate that the greatest augmentation of diastolic aortic pressure occurs at complete occlusion. This condition however is not desirable, from the point of view of afterload reduction, although there have been cases where occlusion up to 95 percent have been shown to give good hemodynamic results. Balloon configuration and its properties are also important. Nonuniform inflation characteristics can cause preferential inflation at the terminal segments of the balloon, resulting in ineffective volume displacement and pressure augmentation. Multiple segment chamber balloons have been designed to eliminate this by causing inflation to proceed from the distal end to the proximal end (closer to the heart). This tends to increase mean diastolic pressure in the region of the coronary arteries and augments coronary perfusion.

The rates of rise and fall of balloon inflation and deflation have been shown both theoretically and experimentally to be crucial determinants of IABP performance (Li *et al.*, 1984). They result from the density and viscosity of the driving gas, and the pressure of the gas source. The three primary driving gases commonly that have been used are helium (He), nitrogen (N_2), and carbon dioxide (CO_2). The use of nitrogen has been commonplace until its replacement by helium. Carbon dioxide was used because of its greater solubility and reduced risk of gas embolism in the event of leakage. Helium use leads to faster rise and fall times. The timing of IABP relative to the diastolic phase of the cardiac cycle is also very important. Experiments performed on dogs verified theoretical predictions on these timing effects (Li *et al.*, 1984; Zelano *et al.*, 1985). It appears that the optimal inflation time is a time period just prior to the aortic valve closure or the dicrotic notch on the pressure tracing. A short delay is necessary to take into account the balloon rise time and the finite propagation time of the pressure pulse in the aorta.

Enhancement of cardiac output and mean diastolic pressure at greatly reduced systolic loading and tension time index values can be achieved. Regional contractile properties in the normal and ischemic border zones are also improved (Fig. 9.5.2). Early inflation will decrease cardiac output and increase myocardial oxygen consumption through an increase in tension-time index. Late inflation will result in a lowering of mean diastolic pressure and a decrease in cardiac output.

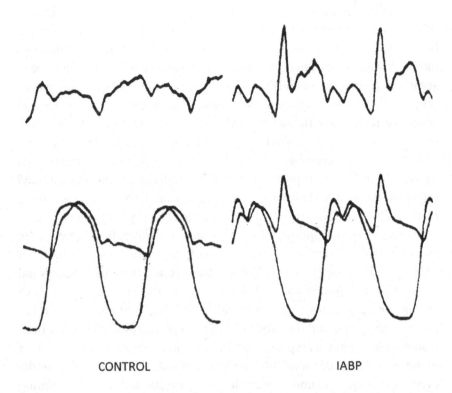

CONTROL   IABP

Fig. 9.5.2: Intra-aortic balloon pump (IABP) efficacy on coronary blood flow. Balloon mounted on a catheter is inserted into the descending thoracic aorta. It is deflated during systolic ejection and inflated after aortic valve closure. Experiment illustrates normal inflation (NIF) and normal deflation (NDF) of the balloon when helium (He) is used as the driving gas which is much faster than either air or nitrogen. This allows more accurate timing of the inflation and deflation of the balloon. Left tracings are recorded during Control and right tracings are recorded during IABP. It can be seen that diastolic aortic pressure is significantly augmented. Since it serves as the coronary perfusion pressure, the coronary blood flow is significantly improved (top right tracing).

Since mean diastolic pressure is proportional to coronary blood flow, coronary perfusion can be seriously compromised by improper timing of balloon inflation. The time of deflation may vary depending upon the desired hemodynamic effects. To minimize end diastolic aortic pressure, it is necessary to deflate the balloon prior to ventricular ejection taking into account the fall time of the gas in the balloon. Ideally, deflation should be timed such that the minimum of the diastolic pressure coincides with the onset of ventricular ejection. This will also minimize ventricular afterload.

Both theoretical and experimental studies have shown that late deflation can increase coronary blood flow and stroke volume substantially. This is particularly beneficial to a failing heart with low cardiac output. But late deflation will also increase the load on the heart during ejection, hence increasing myocardial oxygen consumption. An appropriate compromise would be to produce the maximum increase in mean diastolic pressure and coronary perfusion from systolic augumentation (late deflation) and at the same time keep afterload low.

Deflation bordering on isovolumetric systole seems to be the best choice. This choice tends to maximize the oxygen supply to demand ratio as well as cardiac efficiency, which is defined as the ratio of external work (stroke volume × mean arterial pressure) to myocardial oxygen consumption. It is clear that the duration of the inflation-deflation interval is critical to the ability of an IABP to maximize coronary perfusion and to reduce the work requirements of the failing left ventricle. While timing and inflation-deflation rates are important determinants of IABP performance, other hemodynamic factors can also exert their influences. These include the pressure-diameter relationship of the aorta, peripheral resistance, heart rate, the severity of heart failure and neural-humoral interactions. For instance, a pressure increase will signal the baroreceptor reflexes to alter heart rate. The combined effects of increased balloon occlusion and heart rate at lower pressure enhance augmentation of mean diastolic pressure. The IABP cannot physically pump blood like a cardiac bypass device, and must rely on the heart to perform the necessary work. Thus the severity of heart failure is also a critical determinant of the beneficial effects of IABP.

9.5.3 *Optimization of Intra-Aortic Balloon Pumping: Modeling Aspects*

Modeling studies are useful in providing detailed parameter analyses and to obtain specific predictions which yield quantitative information regarding the interaction of IABP with the cardiovascular system. Some investigators have employed a windkessel model of the vascular system, with a flow source model of the left ventricle, to explain observed changes in left ventricular pressure and aortic flow during IABP using derived mathematical relationships. Others have calculated the relative ventricular work and aortic input impedance as a function of device phasing for the fundamental frequency components and showed that these parameters were minimized when the fundamental components of aortic pressure and flow had a phase difference of 180° (Jaron *et al.*, 1983). Changes in the timing were shown to increase impedance and ventricular work which could limit cardiac output and overload an already weakened heart.

Several investigators have studied the ability of IABP to augment hemodynamic performance dependence on cardiac state. No single combination of device timing variables can simultaneously achieve the best improvement for all hemodynamic parameters considered. Nerz *et al.* (1979) and Cui *et al.* (1990) using a time-varying compliance model of the left ventricle and an arterial system model, studied timing, pumping rate, balloon placement in the aorta, and device stroke volume. They indicated that increasing device pumping rate or rise and fall time of the pumping pulse caused a greater increase in coronary blood flow and cardiac output with a greater decrease in aortic end diastolic pressure. Additional increases in coronary and aortic flows could be obtained when termination of the device pulse occurred past end diastole. The overall improvement in hemodynamic parameters was greater for larger balloon volumes. Balloon inflation at the beginning of end systole was most effective in enhancing hemodynamic parameters. Others have shown that additional increases in coronary and aortic flows can be obtained at the expense of systolic loading with balloon deflation later than end diastole. Some of these model predictions have been verified in experimental animal studies by Li *et al.* (1984) Model studies generally can adequately predict short-term effects of IABP on the cardiovascular system (Dai and Li, 1995). But the long-term effects on the cardiovascular system will have to include physiological control aspects.

9.5.4 *Optimization of Intra-Aortic Balloon Pumping: Control Aspects*

A real-time closed loop control scheme for IABP is necessary because of the heart rate changes and the changes in the physiological state of the cardiovascular system. Dynamic timing adjustments are therefore essential. Dynamic control of the assisted circulation can be performed by, for instance, the utilization of state variable analysis and a conjugate gradient optimization method. The chosen state variables can be the fundamental components and phases of aortic pressure and flow with a constraint for pressure and flow to return to normal. It is obvious that the constraint necessity is for the fundamental components of aortic pressure and flow to be 180 degrees out of phase. This allows maximal coronary perfusion due to aortic diastolic pressure augmentation. A performance index of normalized left ventricular power can then be used to assess the efficacy of counterpulsation.

IABP efficacy is dependent on selected performance indices that are implemented based on the control algorithms. These also need to operate in real-time for practical purposes. These indices should be evaluated on a beat to beat basis and attempts made to either minimize or maximize each index by adjusting balloon timing. Clark *et al.* (1973) developed a closed-loop control scheme to maximize a weighted performance index comprised of mean systolic pressure, mean diastolic pressure, and end diastolic pressure to optimize IABP performance. The algorithm was implemented on both mini- and microcomputers. Timing was controlled using a regression equation to predict the systolic time interval (STI) from the measured heart rate. The algorithm gave reasonable results. Other schemes and computer-based controller have also been applied, based on weighted indices, such as coronary blood flow, tension time index, end diastolic pressure, left ventricular stroke work, and cardiac output, as well as left ventricular viability ratio and endocardial viability ratio, to assess pumping efficacy.

Earlier, we developed a closed loop model of the cardiovascular system in order to evaluate the most suitable control variables for mechanical assistance (Puri *et al.*, 1982). The model assumes that the heart operates on the Frank-Starling mechanism and includes the carotid sinus baroreceptor control. Their results showed that heart rate and left atrial pressure (LAP) were the most sensitive parameters for the control of assistance, and that the extent of assistance is dependent on the severity of heart failure. The choice of the performance index, as well as the weighting factors, is critical in determining IABP efficacy. There is no totally automated system that presently exists clinically for closed-loop control of cardiac assistance. To arrive at this goal it was shown that model studies are important, because they predict either the open-loop or closed-loop quantitative behavior of hemodynamic parameters.

A microprocessor-based controller to implement real-time automation of pump time using an IABP was developed by Zelano *et al.* (1985, 1990). The system sensed atrial P-waves, R-waves, and second heart sounds, and operated in an open loop mode. The results of experiments on dogs with this device indicate that automatic control of IABP in an open loop mode yields equivalent increases in cardiac output, coronary blood flow, with reduced resistance, and decreases in end diastolic pressure and ventricular oxygen consumption when compared to normal control adjustment by a certified balloon pump technician. A closed-loop control algorithm however would be more desirable.

Improvement in the dynamics of the assisted circulation can be valuable once the design of assist devices is refined and the control strategies are better defined. To this end, the understanding of the dynamics of the natural vascular system and its interaction with the heart is a necessary step to the appreciation of the overall function of the circulation.

Bibliography

Altman, P.L. and Dittmer, D.S. *Biology Data Book*. FASEB, Besthesda, 1961.

Anliker, M., Histand, M.B. and Ogden, E. Dispersion and attenuation of small artificial pressure waves in the canine aorta. *Circ. Res.* 23:539-551, 1968.

Anliker, M., Wells, M.K. and Ogden E. The transmission characteristics of large and small pressure waves in the abdominal vena cava. *IEEE Trans. Biomed. Eng.* BME-16:262-273, 1969.

Aoki, T. and Ku, D.N. Collapse of diseased arteries with eccentric cross section. *J. Biomech. Eng.* 26:2:133–42, 1993.

Atlas, G.M. and Li, J.K-J. Brachial artery differential characteristic impedance: contributions from changes in Young modulus and diameter. *Cardiovasc. Eng.* 9:11-17, 2009.

Arntzenius, A.C. The Importance of Pulsations. *Proc. Cardiovasc. System Dynam. Soc Conf.*, Philadelphia, 1976.

Attinger, E.O. *Pulsatile Blood Flow*. McGraw-Hill, New York, 1964.

Bailie, J.A. On the dispersion of waves in fluid-filled cylinders of slightly elliptical cross-section. *J. Biomech.* 5:165, 1972.

Benchimol, A. *Noninvasive Diagnostic Techniques in Cardiology*. Williams & Wilkins, Baltimore, 1981.

Berger, D., Li, J.K-J., Laskey, W.K. and Noordergraaf, A. Repeated reflection of waves in the systemic arterial system. *Am. J. Physiol.* (*Heart & Circ. Physiol.* 33) 264:H269-281, 1993.

Berger, D.S., Li, J. K-J. Temporal relationship between left ventricular and arterial system elastances. *IEEE Trans. Biomed. Eng.* BME-39: 404-410, 1992.

Bevir, M. Sensitivity of electromagnetic velocity probes. *Phys. Med. Biol.* 16:229-232, 1971.

Boccalon, H., Candelon, B., Puel, P., Enjalbert, A., and Doll, H. Assessment of pulsatile blood flow by a noninvasive electromagnetic device. *In Noninvasive Cardiovascular Diagnosis*, ed. E.B. Dietlifich, pp. 231-240. University Park Press, Baltimore, 1978.

Brower, R.W. and Noordergraaf, A. Pressure-flow characteristics of collapsible tubes: A reconciliation of seemingly contradictory results. *Ann. Biomed. Eng.* 1:333, 1973.

Brower, R.W. and Scholten, C. Experimental evidence on the mechanism for the instability of flow in collapsible vessels. *Med. Biol. Eng.* 13:839, 1975.

Brutsaert, D.L. The force-velocity-time interrelation of cardiac muscle. In: *The Physical Basis of Starling's Law of the Heart*, pp. 155-175. Eds. R. Porter and D.W. Fitzsimons, Elsevier, Amsterdam, 1974.

Caro, C.G., Pedley, T.J., Schroter, R.C. and Seed, W.A. *The Mechanics of the Circulation.* Oxford Univ. Press, Oxford, 1978.

Caro, C.G. Discovery of the role of wall shear in atherosclerosis. *Arterioscler. Thromb. Vasc. Biol.* 29:158-161, 2009.

Chaveau, A. and Marey, E. Appareils et experiences cardiographiques. Demonstration nouvelle de mechanisms des mouvements du coeur par l'emploi des instruments enregistreurs a indications continues. *Mem. Acad. Med.* 26: 268, 1863.

Chirinos, J.A., Rietzschel, E.R., Shiva-Kumar, P., Buyzere M.L., Zamani, P., Clasessens, T., Geraci, S., Konda, P., De Bacquer, D., Akers, S.R., Gillebert, T.C. and Segers, P. Effective arterial elastance is insensitive to pulsatile arterial load. *Hypertension.* 64:1022-1031, 2014.

Clark, J.W., Kane, G.R. and Bourland, H.M.. On the feasibility of closed loop control of intra aortic balloon pumping. *IEEE Trans. Biomed. Eng.*, BME-20:404, 1973.

Cox, R.H. and Pace, J.B. Pressure-flow relations in the vessels of the canine aortic arch. *Am. J. Physiol. 228:* 1-10, 1975.

Cox, R.H. Pressure dependence of the mechanical properties of arteries in vivo. *Am. J. Physiol.* 229:1371-1375, 1975.

Craim, D., Graf, S.N., Armentano, R.L. and Barra, J.G. Vascular smooth muscle activation improves aortic compliance with respect to mechanical loading. *Cardiovasc. Eng. Tech.*, 3:80-87, 2012.

Cui, T., Welkowitz, W., Li, J.K-J., Petrucelli, S. and Spotnitz, A. A novel mechanical cardiac assist device for reversing left ventricular failure. *Trans. Am. Soc. Artif. Internal Organs*, 36:401-404, 1990.

Dai, J.-W. and Li, J.K-J. Aortic impedance alteration on the response of single segment intra-aortic balloon pumping: A model-based analysis. *Ann. Biomed. Eng.*, 23:S40, 1995.

DeBakey, M.E., Lawrie, G.M. and Glaeser, D.H. Patterns of atherosclerosis and their surgical significance. *Ann. Surg.*, 201, 115-131, 1985.

Drzewiecki, G., Field, S., Mubarak, I. and Li, J.K-J. Effect of vascular growth pattern on lumen area and compliance using a novel pressure-area model for collapsible vessels. *Am. J. Physiol. (Heart & Circ. Physiol.)*, 273:H2030-2043, 1997.

Drzewiecki, G.M., Melbin, J. and Noordergraaf, A. Noninvasive blood pressure recording and the genesis of Korotkoff sound. Ch.8, *Handbook of Bioengineering*, Eds.: R. Skalak and S. Chien. New York: McGraw-Hill, 1987.

Drzewiecki, G.M., Melbin, J. and Noordergraaf, A. Arterial tonometry: Review and analysis. *J. Biomech.* 16: 141-152, 1983.

Fawcett, D.W. *A Textbook of Histology.* Chapman & Hill, New York, 1994.

Frank, O. Die Grundform des arteriellen pulses. *Z. Biol.* 37:483-526, 1899.

Friedman, M.R. and L.W. Ehrlich. Numerical simulation of aortic bifurcation flows: The effect of flow divider curvature. *J. Biomech.* 17:881-888, 1984.

Fronek, A. and V. Ganz. Measurement of flow in single vessels including cardiac output by local thermodilution. *Circ. Res.* 8:175, 1960.

Fung, Y.C. *Biomechanics: Circulation.* Springer-Verlag, New York, 1997.

Galilei, G. *Dialogues Concerning Two New Sciences.* 1637. Translated version (H. Crew and A. DeSalvio): Macmillan, New York, 1914.

Ganz, W. R., Donoso, R., Marcus, H.S., Forrester, J.S. and Swan, H.J.C. A new technique for measurement of cardiac output by thermodiluation. *Am. J. Cardiol.* 27:392-396, 1971.

Geddes, L.A. *Cardiovascular Devices and Their Applications.* Wiley, New York, 1984.

Goto, M., Yanaka, M., Yosifumi, W., Hiramatsu, O., Ogasawara, Y., Tsujioka, K. and Kajiya, F. Analysis of phasic blood flow velocity in atrial coronary arteries and veins by laser Doppler method. *Proc. 9th Cardiovasc. System Dynam. Conf.,* pp.125-128, 1988.

Green, H.D. Circulatory system: Physical principles. In: *Medical Physics* 2, Ed. O. Glasser, Year Book Publishers, New York, 1950.

Hagenbach, E. Uber die Bestimming der Sahigkeit einer Flussigkeit durch den Ausfluss aus Rohren. *Ann. Der Physik.* 109:385-426, 1860.

Hales, S. *Statical Essays Containing Haemostaticks.* London, 1733.

Hartley, C.J., Reddy, A.K., Madala, S., Michael, L.H., Entman, M.L. and Taffet, G.E. Doppler estimation of reduced coronary flow reserve in mice with pressure overload cardiac hypertrophy. *Ultrasound Med. Biol.* 34: 892–901, 2008.

Hartley, C.J., Michael, L.H. and Entman, M.L. Noninvasive measurement of ascending aortic blood velocity in mice. *Am. J. Physiol.* 268:H499-505, 1995.

Harvey, W. *De Motu Cordis.* London, 1628.

Holt, J.P. Flow through collapsible tubes and through in situ veins. *IEEE Trans. Biomed. Eng.* BME-16: 274-283, 1969.

Huo, Y., Finet, G., Lefevre, T., Louvard, Y., Moussa, I. and Kassab, G.S. Which diameter and angle rule provides optimal flow patterns in a coronary bifurcation? *J. Biomech.* 45:1273-1279, 2012.

Intaglietta, M., Parvula, R.F. and Thompkins, W.R. Pressure measurements in the Mammalian microvasculature. *Microvasc. Res.* 2: 212-220, 1970.

Intaglietta, M., Richardson, D.R. and Thompkins, W.R. Blood pressure, flow, and elastic properties in microvessels of cat omentum. *Am. J. Physiol.* 221:922-928, 1971.

Ishihara, M., Sato H., Tateishi H., Uchida T. and Dote K. Intraaortic balloon pumping as the postangioplasty strategy in acute myocardial infarction. *Am. Heart J.* 122:385-389, 1991.

Jacobs, L.A., Klopp, E.H., Seamore, W., Topaz, S.R. and Gott, V.L. Improved organ functions during cardiac bypass with a roller pump modified to deliver pulsatile flow. *J. Thorac. Cardio. Surg.* 58:703-712, 1969.

Jager, G.N., Westerhof, N. and Noordergraaf, A. Oscillatory flow impedance in electrical analog of arterial system. *Circ. Res.* 16:121-133, 1965.

Jaron, D., Moore, T. and He, P. Theoretical considerations regarding the optimization of cardiac assistance by intraaortic balloon pumping. *IEEE Trans. Biomed. Eng.*, BME-30:117, 1983.

Kalmanson, D. and Veyrat, C. Clinical aspects of venous return: A velocimetric approach to a new system dynamic concept. In: *Cardiovascular System Dynamics*, eds. J. Baan, A. Noordergraaf and J. Raines, pp. 297, MIT Press, 1978.

Karreman, G. Some contributions to the mathematical biology of blood circulation. Reflections of pressure wave in the arterial system. *Bull. Math. Biophys.* 14:327-350, 1952.

Kassab, G.S., Rider, C.A., Tang, N.J., Fung, Y.C. Morphometry of pig coronary arterial trees. *Am. J. Physiol. (Heart & Circ.)* 265:H350–H365, 1993.

Kaya, M. and Li, J.K-J. Modeling aspects of hemorrhage and hemodilution. *Proc. 28th NE Bioeng. Conf.*, pp. 177-178, 2002.

Kerkhof, P.L.M., Li, J.K-J. and Kresh, J.Y. An analytical expression for the regulation of ventricular volume in the normal and diseased Heart. *Cardiovasc. Eng.* 2:37-48, 2002.

Kerkhof, P.L.M., Li, J.K-J. and Heyndrix, H.R. Effect of arterial elastance and arterial compliance in heart failure patients with preserved ejection fraction. *Proc. 36th IEEE Eng. Med. Biol. Conf.*, pp. 691-694, 2013.

Kerkhof, P.L.M., Kresh, J.Y., Li, J.K-J. and Heyndrickx, G.R. Left ventricular volume regulation in heart failure with preserved ejection fraction. *Physiol. Report*, 1(2):1-10, 2013.

Kelly, R.P., Tang C-T., Yang, T.-M., Liu, C.-P., Maughan, W.L., Chang, M.-S. and Kass, D. Effective arterial elastance as index of arterial vascular load in humans. *Circ.* 86:513-521, 1992.

Knowleton, F.P. and E.H. Starling. The influence of variations in temperature and blood pressure on the performance of the isolated mammalian heart. *J. Physiol.* 44:206-219, 1912.

Korteweg, D.J. Uber die Fortpflanzungsgeschwindigkeit des Schalles in elastischen Rohren. *Ann. Phys. Chem.* 5:525-537, 1878.

Kresch, E. and Noordergraaf, A. A mathematical model for the pressure-flow relationships in a segment of veins. *IEEE Trans. Biomed. Eng.* 16:296, 1969.

Kresch, E. and Noordergraaf, A. Cross-sectional shape of collapsible tubes. *Biophys. J.* 12:274, 1972.

Lamb, H. On the velocity of sound in a tube as affected by the elasticity of the walls. *Manchester Mem.* 42:1-16, 1898.

Iberall, A.S. Anatomy and steady flow characteristics of the arterial system with an introduction to its pulsatile characteristics. *Math. Biosci.* 1:375-395, 1967.

Lee, J.S. and Skalak T.C. *Microvascular Mechanics*. Springer-Verlag, New York, 1989.

Lee, J.S. and Schmid-Schonbein, G.W. Biomechanics of skeletal muscle capillaries: hemodynamic resistance, endothelial distensibility, and pseudopod formulation. *Ann. Biomed. Eng.* 23:226-246, 1995.

Lee, J.S., Salathe, E.P. and Schmid-Schonbein, G.W. Fluid exchange in skeletal muscle with viscoelastic blood vessels. *Am. J. Physiol.* 253:H1548-H1566, 1987.

Lei, C.Q. and Li, J.K-J. Comparison of time domain and frequency domain assessments of arterial wave reflections. *Proc. 22nd. NE Bioeng. Conf.*, 22:7-8, 1996.

Li, J.K-J. Oxygen cost to work ratio in pressure-loaded ventricle. *Proc. 35th Ann. Conf. Eng. Med. Biol.*, 24, 145, 1982.

Li, J.K-J. Pressure-derived flow: A new method. *IEEE Trans. Biomed. Eng.*, BME-30, 244-246, 1983.

Li, J.K-J. Hemodynamic significance of metabolic turnover rate. *J. Theor. Biol.*, 103:333-338, 1983.

Li, J.K-J. Time domain resolution of forward and reflected waves in the aorta. *IEEE Trans. Biomed. Eng.*, BME-33:783-785, 1986.

Li, J.K-J. Dominance of geometric over elastic factors in pulse transmission through arterial branching. *Bull. Math. Biol.*, 48, 97-103, 1986.

Li, J.K-J. Comparative cardiac mechanics: Laplace's law. *J. Theor. Biol.*, 118, 339-343, 1986.

Li, J.K-J. *Arterial System Dynamics.* New York Univ. Press, 1987.

Li, J.K-J. Regional left ventricular mechanics during myocardial ischemia. In: *Simulation and Modeling of the Cardiac System.* pp. 451-462, Ed. S. Sideman, Martinus Nijhoff Publishers, 1987.

Li, J.K-J. Laminar and turbulent flow in the mammalian aorta: Reynolds number. *J. Theor. Biol.*, 135:409-414, 1988.

Li, J.K-J., Significance of systolic aortic pressure to flow ratio. *Proc. 13th. Internat. Conf. Eng. Med. Biol.*, 13:2043, 1991.

Li, J.K-J. *Comparative Cardiovascular Dynamics of Mammals.* CRC Press, New York, 1996.

Li, J.K.-J. A new description of arterial function: The compliance-pressure loop. *Angiology, J. Vasc. Dis.* 49:543-548, 1998.

Li, J.K-J. Scaling and invariants in cardiovascular biology. In: *Scaling in Biology*, pp. 113-128, eds. J.H. Brown and G.B. West, Oxford Univ. Press, 2000.

Li, J.K-J. *The Arterial Circulation: Physical Principles and Clinical Applications.* Human Press (Springer), New York, 2000.

Li, J.K-J., Van Brummelen, A.G.W. and Noordergraaf, A. Fluid-filled blood pressure measurement systems. *J. Appl. Physiol.* 40: 839-843, 1976.

Li, J.K-J. and Noordergraaf, A. Evaluation of needle-manometer and needle differential-manometer systems in the measurement of pressure differences. *Proc. 3rd NE Bioeng. Conf.* 5: 275-277, 1977.

Li, J.K-J., Melbin, J., Campbell, K.B. and Noordergraaf, A. Evaluation of a three-point pressure method for the determination of arterial transmission characteristics. *J. Biomechanics*, 13, 1023-1029, 1980.

Li, J.K-J., Melbin, J. and Noordergraaf, A. Pulse transmission to vascular beds. *Proc. 33rd ACEMB* 22: 109, 1980.

Li, J.K-J., Melbin, J., Riffle, R.A. and Noordergraaf, A. Pulse wave propagation. *Circ. Res.* 49, 442-452, 1981.

Li, J.K-J., Welkowitz, W., Zelano, J., Molony, D.A., Kostis, J.B., and Mackenzie, J.W. Effects of balloon inflation and deflation rates on global and regional ventricular performance. *Progress Artif. Organs*, 137- 140, 1983.

Li, J.K-J., Welkowitz, W., Zelano, J., Molony, D.A., Kostis, J.B. and Mackenzie, J.W. Intraortic balloon counterpulsation: blood flow increment dependence on inflation interval. *Proc. 6th. Internat. Cardiovascular System Dynamics*, 6:72-75, 1984.

Li, J.K-J., Melbin, J. and Noordergraaf, A. Directional disparity of pulse wave reflections in dog arteries. *Am. J. Physiol. (Heart & Circ. Physiol.)*, 247:H95-99, 1984.

Li, J.K-J. and Kostis, J.B. Aspects determining accurate diagnosis and efficacy of catheterization. *Proc. 1st Int. Congr. Med. Instrument.* A07, 1984.

Li, J.K-J., Cui, T. and Drzewiecki, G. A nonlinear model of the arterial system incorporating a pressure-dependent compliance. *IEEE Trans. Biomed. Eng.*, BME-37:673-678, 1990.

Li, J.K-J. and Zhu Y. Arterial compliance and its pressure dependence in hypertension and vasodilation. *Angiology, J. Vasc. Diseas.* 45:113-117, 1994.

Li, J.K-J., McMahon, R., Singh, M., Zhu, Y., Amory, D., Drzewiecki, G. and O'Hara, D.A. Noninvasive pulse wave velocity and apparent phase velocity in normal and hypertensive subjects. *J. Cardiovas. Diagn. Procedures*, 13:31-36, 1996.

Li, J.K-J., Zhu, Y. and Geipel, P.S. Pulse pressure, arterial compliance and wave reflection under differential vasoactive and mechanical loading. *Cardiovasc. Eng.* 10:170-175, 2010.

Li, J.K-J., Wang, T. and Zhang, H. Rapid noninvasive continuous monitoring of oxygenation in cerebral ischemia and hypoxia. *Cardiovasc. Eng.* 10:213-217, 2010.

Li, J.K-J. and Atlas, A. Left ventricle–arterial system interaction in heart failure. *Clinical Medicine Insights: Cardiology, Suppl.* 93-99, 2015.

Li, J.K-J., Zhu Y. and Noordergraaf, A. A comparative approach to analysis and modeling of cardiovascular function. *Molecular, Cellular, and Tissue Engineering, in Biomedical Engineering Handbook*, 4th ed. Chapter 26, pp. 26:1-12, Ed. J.D. Bronzino, D.R. Peterson, CRC Press, Boca Raton, London, New York, 2015.

Liao, J., Li, J.K-J. and Metaxas, D. Characterization of time-varying properties and regional strains in myocardial ischemia. *Cardiovasc. Eng.* 3:109-116, 2003.

Ling, S.C. Atabek, H.B., Letzing, W.G. and Patel, D.J. Nonlinear analysis of aortic flow in living dogs. *Circ. Res.* 33:198-212, 1973.

MacFadyen, R.J., Lees, K.R. and Reid, J.L. Double blind controlled study of low dose intravenous perindoprilat or enalaprilat infusion in elderly patients with heart failure. *Br Heart J.* 69:293-297, 1993.

MacFadyen, R.J. Looking backwards and moving forwards in the therapy of hypertension. *Therapy* 5:727-730, 2008.

Mates, R.E., Gupta, R.L., Bell, A.C. and Klocke, F.J. Fluid dynamics of coronary artery stenosis. *Circ. Res.* 42:152-162, 1978.

Matonick, J.P. and Li, J.K-J. Noninvasive monitoring of blood pressure during handgrip stress induced vascular reactivity. *Proc. 34th. Assoc. Adv. Med. Instrum.*, 1999.

Matonick, J. and Li, J.K-J. Pressure-dependent and frequency domain characteristics of the systemic arterial system. *Cardiovasc. Eng.* 1:21-29, 2001.

Maughan, W.L., Sunagawa, K., Burkhoff, D. and Sagawa, K. Effect of arterial impedance changes on the end-systolic pressure-volume relation. *Circ. Res.* 54:595-602, 1984.

Mayrovitz, H.N., Wiedeman, M.P. and Noordergraaf A. Analytical characterization of microvascular resistance distribution. *Bull. Math. Biol.* 38:71, 1976.

Mayrovitz, H.N., Wiedeman, M.P. and Noordergraaf, A. Microvascular hemodynamic variations accompanying microvessel dimensional changes. *Microvasc. Res.* 10:322, 1975.

Mayrovitz, H.N. Assessment of human Microvascular Function. In: *Analysis and Assessment of Cardiovascular Function.* pp. 248-273. Eds: G. Drzewiecki and J. K-J. Li, Springer-Verlag, New York, 1998.

McDonald, D.A. *Blood Flow in Arteries.* Arnold, London, 1960, 1974.

Millasseau, S.C., Patel, S.J., Redwood, S.R., Ritter, J.M. and Chowienczyk, P.J. Pressure wave reflection assessed from the peripheral pulse. Is a transfer function necessary? *Hypertension*, 41:1016-1020, 2003.

Mills, C.J. A catheter-tip electromagnetic flow probe. *Phys. Med. Biol.* 11:323-324, 1966.

Moens, A.I. *Die Pulskurve.* Leiden, 1878.

Moreno, A.H. Dynamics of pressure in central veins. In: *Cardiovascular System Dynamics*, eds. J. Baan, A. Noordergraaf and J. Raines, pp. 266, MIT Press, 1978.

Moreno, A.H., Katz, A.I., Gold, L. and Reddy. R.V. Mechanical distension of dog veins and other very thin-walled tubular structures. *Circ. Res.* 27:1069-1079, 1970.

Morgan, B.C., Abel, F.L., Mullins, G.L. and Guntheroth, W.G. Flow patterns in the cavae, pulmonary artery, pulmonary vein and aorta in intact dogs. *Am. J. Physiol.* 210:903, 1966.

Morgan, G.W. and Kiely, J.P. Wave propagation in a viscous liquid contained in a flexible tube. *J. Acoust. Soc. Am.* 26:323-328, 1954.

Mueller, H.S. Role of intra-aortic counterpulsation in cardiogenic shock and acute myocardial infarction. *Cardiol.* 84:168-174, 1994.

Nerz, R., Myerowitz, P.D. and Blackshear, P.L. A simulation of the dynamics of counterpulsation. *J. Biomech. Eng.*, 101:105, 1979.

Nichols, W.W. and O'Rourke, M.F. *McDonald's Blood Flow in Arteries.* 4th. edition, Arnold, London, 1998.

Nichols, W.W., Conti, C.R., Walker, W.E. and Milnor, W.R. Input impedance of the systematic circulation in man. *Circ. Res.* 40: 451-458, 1977.

Nichols, W.W. and McDonald, D.A. Wave velocity in the proximal aorta. *Med. Biol. Eng.* 10: 327-335, 1972.

Noordergraaf, A. *Circulatory System Dynamics.* Academic Press, New York, 1978.

Noordergraaf, A. Hemodynamics. In: *Biological Engineering.* Ed: H.P. Schwan. McGraw-Hill, New York, 1969.

Noordergraaf, A. *Blood in Motion.* Springer, New York, 2011.

Ohman, E.M., Goeroge, B.S., White, C.J., Kern, M.J., Gurbel, P.A., Freeman, R.J., *et al.* Use of aortic counterpulsation to improve sustained coronary artery patency during acute myocardial infarction: Results of a randomized trial. *Circ.* 90:792-299, 1994.

Oka, S. *Cardiovascular Hemorheology.* Cambridge Univ. Press, London, 1981.

Olufsen, M.S., Peskin, C.S., Kim, W.Y., Petersen, E.M., Nadim, A. and Larsen, J. Numerical simulation and experimental validation of blood flow in arteries with structured-tree outflow conditions. *Ann. Biomed. Eng.* 28:1281-1299, 2000.

Patel, A.M., Li, J.K-J., Finegan, B. and McMurtry, M.S. Aortic pressure estimation using blind identification approach on single input multiple output non-linear Wiener systems. *IEEE Trans. Biomed. Eng.*, DOI 10.1109/TBME.2017.2688425, IEEE.

Patel, A.M. and Li, J.K-J. Validation of a novel nonlinear black box Wiener System model for arterial pulse transmission. *Comput. Biol. Med.* 88, 2017. DOI: 10.1016/j.compbiomed.2017.06.020

Perktold, K. and Rappitsch, G. Computer simulation of local blood flow and vessel mechanics in a compliant carotid artery bifurcation model *J. Biomech.*, 28:845–856, 1995.

Permutt, S., Bromberger-Barnea, B. and Bane, H.N.. Alveolar pressure, pulmonary venous pressure, and the vascular waterfall. *Med. Thorac.* 19:239-260, 1962.

Phan, T.S., Khaw, K. and Li, J.K-J. Integrating increased pulse wave velocity and reflections on late systolic ventricular loading and unloading. *J. Am. Soc. Hypertension* 9(4S): e87–e88, 2015.

Phan, T.S., Li, J.K-J., Segers, P. and Chirinos, J.A. Misinterpretation of the determinants of elevated forward wave amplitude inflates the role of the proximal aorta. *J. Am. Heart Assoc., DOI: 10.1161/JAHA.115.003069,* 2016.

Phan, T.S., Li, J.K-J., Segers, P., Koppula, M.R., Akers, S.R., Kuna, S.T., Gislason, T., Pack, A.I. and Chirinos, J.A. Aging is associated with an earlier arrival of reflected waves without a distal shift in reflection sites. *J. Am. Heart Assoc.* 2016; 5:e003733 doi: 10.1161/JAHA.116.003733.

Pierce, W.S. *et al.* Ventricular-assist pumping in patient with cardiogenic shock after cardiac operations. *N. Engl. J. Med.*, 305: 1606-1610, 1981.

Pliskow, B.L., Li, J.K-J., O'Hara, D.A. and Kaya M. A novel approach to modeling acute normovolemic hemodilution. *Comput. Biol. Med.*, 68:155-164, 2016.

Puri, N. N., Li, J.K-J., Fich, S. and Welkowitz, W. Control system for circulatory assist devices: Determination of suitable control variables. *Trans. Am. Soc. Artif. Intern. Organs,* 28:127-132, 1982.

Robard, S. Autoregulation in encapsulated, passive, soft-walled vessels. *Am. Heart J.* 65:648, 1963.

Roberts, V.C. *Blood Flow Measurements.* Williams and Wilkins, Baltimore, 1972.

Rosen, R. *Optimality Principles in Biology.* Butterworth, London, 1967.

Rushmer, R.F. *Structure and Function of the Cardiovascular System.* Saunders, Philadelphia, 1972.

Salotto, A., Muscarella, L.F., Melbin, J., Li, J.K-J. and Noordergraaf, A. Pressure pulse transmission into vascular beds. *Microvasc. Res.* 32:152-163, 1986.

Schreiner, W., Karch, R., Neumann, F. and Neumann, M. Constrained constructive optimization of arterial tree models. pp. 145-165. In: Brown, J.H. and G.B. West. *Scaling in Biology.* Oxford University Press, 2000.

Shung, K.K. *Diagnostic Ultrasound: Imaging and Blood Flow Measurements.* CRC Press, Boca Raton, 2005.

Smaje, L., Zweifach, B.W. and Intaglietta, M. Micropressures and capillary filtration coefficients in single vessels of the cremaster muscle of the rat. *Microvasc. Res.* 2:96-110, 1970.

Somlyo, A.P. and Somlyo, A.V. Vascular smooth muscle, I. Normal structure, pathology, biochemistry and biophysics. *Pharm. Rev.* 20:197-272, 1968.

Srichai, M.B., Lim, R.P., Wong, S. and Lee., V.S Cardiovascular applications of phase contrast MRI. *Am. J. Radiol.* 192:662-675, 2009.

Stahl, W.R. Similarity analysis of biological systems. *Persp. Biol. Med.,* 6:291, 1963.

Starling, M.R. Left ventricular-arterial coupling relations in the normal human heart. *Am. Heart J.* 125:1659-1666, 1993.

Suga, H., Sagawa, K. and Shoukas, A. Load independence of the instantaneous pressure-volume ratio of the canine left ventricle and effects of epinephrine and heart rate on the ratio, *Circ. Res.* 32:314-322, 1973.

Sugi, H. and Pollack, G.H. *Mechanism of Sliding Muscle Contraction.* Plenum Press, New York, 1993.

Sunagawa, K., Maughan, W.L., Burkhoff, D. and Sagawa, K. Left ventricular interaction with arterial load studied in isolated canine left ventricle. *Am. J. Physiol.* 265: H773-780, 1983.

Tarbell, J.M., Shi, J.-D., Dunn, J. and Jo, H. Fluid mechanics, arterial disease and gene expression. *Ann. Rev Fluid Mech.* 46:591-614, 2014.

Thubrikar, M.J. and Robicsec, S. Pressure-induced arterial wall stress and atherosclerosis. *Ann. Thorac. Surg.* 59:1594-1603, 1995.

Van Brummelen, A.G.W. Some digital computer applications to hemodynamics. Ph.D. dissertation, University of Utrecht, The Netherlands, 1961.

Van den Bos, G.C., Westerhof, N. and Randall, O.S. Pulse wave reflection: Can it explain the differences between systemic and pulmonary pressure and flow waves? *Circ. Res.* 51:470-485, 1982.

Waksman, R., Weiss, A.T., Gotsman, M.S.a and Hasin Y. Intra-aortic balloon counterpulsation improves survival in cardiogenic shock complicating acute myocardial infarction. *Eur. Heart J.* 14:71-74, 1993.

Wang, R., Pan, Q., Kuebler, W., Li, J.K-J., Pries, A.R. and Ning, G. Modeling of pulsatile flow-dependent nitric oxide regulation in a realistic microvascular network. *Microvasc. Res.* 113:40-49, 2017.

Weizsacker, H.W. and Pascal, K. Anisotropic passive properties of blood vessel walls. In: *Cardiovascular System Dynamics: Models and Measurements*, pp. 347-362. Eds. T. Kenner, R. Busse, H. Hinghofer-Szalkay, Plenum, 1982.

Wells, S.M., Langeille, B.L. and Adamson, S.L. In vivo and in vitro mechanical properties of the sheep in thoracic aorta in the perinatal period and adulthood. *Am. J. Physiol.* 274:H1749-H1760, 1998.

Westerhof, N. and Noordergraaf, A. Arterial viscoelasticity: A generalized model. *J. Biomech.* 3:357-379, 1970.

Westerhof, N., Bosman, F., DeVries, C.J., and Noordergraaf, A. Analog studies of the human systemic arterial tree. *J. Biomech.* 2:121-143, 1969.

Wiederhielm, C.A., Woodbury, J.W., Kirk, S. and Rushmer, R.F. Pulsatile pressure in microcirculation of the frog's mesentery. *Am. J. Physiol.* 207:173-176, 1964.

Wilkins, H., Regdson, W., and Hoffmeister, F.S. The physiological importance of pulsatile blood flow. *New Engl. J. Med.* 267:443-445, 1967.

Womersley, J.R. The mathematical analysis of the arterial circulation in a state of oscillatory motion. *WADC Tech. Rept.* WADC-TR56-614, 1957.

Wyatt, D.G. Blood flow and blood velocity measurement in vivo by electromagnetic induction. *Med. Biol. Eng. Comput.* 22:193-211, 1984.

Yada, T., Hiramatsu, O., Kimura, A., Goto, M., Ogasawaray, Y., Tsujioka, K., Yamamori, S., Ohno, K., Hosaka, H. and Kajiya, F. In vivo observation of subendocardial microvessels of the beating porcine heart using a needle-probe videomicroscope with a CCD camera. *Circ. Res.* 72:939-946, 1993.

Yao, S.T. and Pearce, W.H. The use of noninvasive tests in peripheral vascular disease: Current status. In: *Modern Vascular Surgery*, ed. J.B. Chang, Vol. 4, pp. 49-65, PMA Publishing, California, 1991.

Zamir, M. Vascular system of the human heart: Some branching and scaling issues. In: Brown, J.H. and G.B. West. *Scaling in Biology*. Oxford University Press, 2000.

Zelano, J., Li, J.K-J., Welkowitz, W., Molony, D.A., Kostis, J. and Mackenzie, J. Real-time automation of intra-aortic balloon pumping. *Progr. Artif. Organs*, 85:491-499, 1985.

Zelano, J.A., Li, J.K-J. and Welkowitz, W. A closed loop control scheme for intra-aortic balloon pumping. *IEEE Trans. Biomed. Eng.* BME-37:182-192, 1990.

Zhang, H. and Li, J.K-J A Novel wave reflection model of the human arterial system." *Cardiovasc. Eng.* 9:39-48, 2009.

Zhu, Y. *Computer Based Analysis of Systolic/Diastolic Left Ventricular Function and Pressure-Dependent Arterial Compliance.* Ph.D. dissertation, Rutgers University, NJ, 1996.

Zweifach, B.W. and Lipowsky, H.H. Quantitative studies of microcirculatory structure and function. III. Microvascular hemodynamics of cat mesentery and rabbit omentum. *Circ. Res.* 41:380-390, 1977.

Zweifach, B.W. Quantitative studies of microcirculatory structure and functions. I. Analysis of pressure distribution in the terminal vascular bed. *Circ. Res.* 34:858-866, 1974.

Index

A

abdominal aorta, 100
adventitia, 24
afterload reduction, 255
afterload, 90, 231
allometry, 22
Alternative Starling's Curve, 238
anisotropic properties, 26, 30, 234
anisotropy, 29
aorta, 80, 89
aortic arch, 138
aortic flow, 231, 240
aortic pressure waveform, 60
aortic pressure, 63
aortic valve, 82, 229
aorto-iliac junction, 19, 159
apparent phase constant, 95
apparent phase velocity, 96–97
apparent propagation constant, 94, 97
area ratio, 21, 23, 154, 156,
    158–159
arterial compliance, 103, 125, 128,
    130, 132–133, 249
arterial elastance, 241–243
arterioles, 113
ascending aortic pressure, 108
atherosclerosis, 9, 149–151
attenuation coefficient, 91, 100,
    200
attenuation, 82, 122, 181–182
augmentation index, 111–112

augmented pressure, 83
auscultation method, 214
autonomic nervous system, 38

B

baroreceptors, 38–40
Bernouilli's equation, 11, 71, 174
bifurcation, 138, 144–148, 153–154
biological scaling, 46
blood flow, 44, 48
blood plasma, 31–32
blood pressure waveforms, 5–6, 57,
    62, 80, 205, 218, 212
blood pressure, 5, 44
blood volume, 13, 35–36
blood-wall interactions, 120
body size, 37, 78, 187
brachial artery, 89, 217
brachial pulse, 97
brachial, 206
branching geometry, 144
branching morphology, 144–145
branching structures, 139–140, 187
branching topology, 137
branching, 112, 163
Buckingham's Pi-theorem, 43,
    45–46

C

capillaries, 185–186, 188, 190
cardiac assist device, 14

cardiac contractility, 74, 239, 243
cardiac contraction, 14, 74, 229
cardiac muscle segment length, 230
cardiac output, 19–20, 170, 184, 238,
    242, 252, 255
carotid arteries, 19, 23, 90, 138, 144
carotid pulse, 97
carotid sinus, 39–40
carotid-to-femoral pulse wave
    velocity, 94
carotid-to-radial pulse wave velocity,
    94
catheterization, 6
catheter-manometer systems,
    209–210
catheter-tip pressure transducer, 80,
    212–213
centerline velocity, 68, 116
central aortic pressure, 97, 135
central ischemic zone, 253
central venous pressure, 170, 172
central venous pulses, 171
characteristic impedance, 86–89,
    102, 109, 129, 153–154
chemoreceptors, 38, 40
circumferential stresses, 217
closed loop model, 259
closed-loop control, 260
collagen, 24, 26, 29–30, 41, 100, 120
collapse tube, 182
collapse, 170
collapsibility, 169, 171
collapsible tube, 176, 178
collapsible vessel, 173, 177
collapsible, 175
compliance, 30, 48, 87, 89, 124, 126,
    167, 172, 194, 207
compliance-pressure loops, 136
constrained constructive
    optimization, 142–143
contractility, 235, 241
coronary arteries, 3, 18, 139, 150,
    231, 251

coronary blood flow, 257–258
creep, 51, 55
cube law, 162, 165

D
damping factors, 210–211
damping, 82, 91, 101, 122
diastole, 2
diastolic aortic pressure decay, 127
diastolic filling, 231
diastolic pressure, 79–80, 214, 254
dimensional analysis, 43, 46
dimensional matrix, 45–46
distensibility of capillaries, 193
distensibility, 194, 201
distributed model, 11, 107, 201
Doppler ultrasound, 223
Doppler, 221–222
dye dilution, 224
dynamic elastic modulus, 53–54

E
eccentricity, 179
effective reflection site, 113
ejection fraction, 235, 238–239,
    248–249
elastic laminae, 24
elastic modulus, 53–54
elastic nonuniformities, 82, 112
elastic properties, 89, 156
elastin, 24, 26, 29, 41, 100, 120
electrical analog, 128
electromagnetic flow probe, 80, 221
electromagnetic flowmeter, 219–220
end-diastole, 82
end-diastolic volume, 235, 237, 239
endothelial cells, 24, 187
endothelial NO production, 204
endothelial, 120
endothelium, 183, 188
end-systole, 82
end-systolic pressure-volume
    relation, 240

end-systolic volume, 235
energy dissipation, 9
exchange vessels, 20
external work (EW) of the heart, 237

F
Fahraeus-Lindqvist effect, 191, 201
femoral arteries, 99, 206
femoral artery, 19
femoral artery, 19, 84, 92, 101
filling pressure, 170, 239
flow acceleration, 74
flow limitation, 175
flow velocity, 175
flow waveforms, 12, 141, 147, 220
flow-limiting, 174
fluid-filled blood pressure
    measurement systems, 206, 212
fluid-filled catheter, 205
fluid-filled catheter-manometer
    system, 211
fluid-tissue interface, 120
fluid-wall interaction, 114, 117
foot-to-foot velocity, 91–93, 182
force-velocity-length relations, 246
force-velocity-length, 235
four-element model, 129
Fourier analysis, 56, 84
Fourier series, 57, 59
Frank-Starling, 237
frequency responses, 207–208,
    211–212, 217

G
Galen, 2
Galileo Galilei, 2
geometric nonuniformities, 10, 79,
    81–82
geometric taper, 19, 21–23

H
Hales, 6
harmonic component, 59–60, 63, 85

harmonic contents, 84
heart failure with preserved ejection
    fraction, 14
heart failure, 248, 254, 257
heart valves, 3, 17
heart-arterial system interaction, 83
Hematocrit, 35
hemodynamics, 79
hemoglobin, 32–34
HFpEF, 248–250
HFrEF, 248–250
Hill Model, 234
Hooke's law of elasticity, 5, 25
Hooke's law, 28, 50
hypertension, 9, 26, 135–136, 166,
    237, 245
hypertensive, 97–98, 140
hypertrophy, 237
hypoxia, 34–35
hysteresis, 51–53

I
impedance, 177–178
incompressible, 29, 47, 50, 118
incremental elastic modulus, 53
indicator dilution techniques, 36
inflection pressure, 83
input impedance, 84, 86, 90, 96, 129
interaction of the heart and the
    arterial system, 9
intra-aortic balloon pump (*see also*
    IABP), 14, 250–252, 255–258,
    260
isotropic, 29, 121
isotropy, 25–26
isovolumic contraction, 234
isovolumic phases, 233

J
jugular pressure pulse, 173
jugular pressure, 172
jugular vein, 171
jugular venous pulse, 172

K
kinetic energy, 70
Korotkoff sound, 213, 215–216

L
Lamb mode velocity, 117
Lame equation, 50
laminar flow, 67, 77
Laplace's law, 28, 45, 50
late systolic loading, 245
left ventricle, 2, 15, 82, 90
left ventricular assist devices
(*see also* LVAD), 253–254
left ventricular diastolic pressure,
231
left ventricular pressure, 82,
229–231, 240
Leonardo da Vinci, 3
local reflection coefficient, 152,
155–156, 159–160
local wave reflection, 153
LV-AS coupling, 249–250

M
mammalian species, 10, 15, 80
mammals, 187, 238
maximal elastance, 243
maximum elastance, 240, 244
maximum velocity of cardiac muscle
shortening, 246
maximum velocity of shortening,
240
Maxwell model, 55, 123
Maxwell, 56
mechanism, 237
mechanoreceptors, 38
microcirculation, 183–184, 187
model, 204
modeling, 114, 201, 258
Moens-Korteweg formula, 25, 93,
116–117
Moens-Korteweg relation, 156
multiple reflection, 110, 113

Murray's law, 162–163, 165–166
myocardial oxygen consumption, 1,
255, 257

N
Navier-Stokes equations, 11, 65,
118–119, 121, 123, 130, 136, 147
near infrared, 219
near-infrared oxygenation
monitoring, 34
needle-pressure transducer system,
206
Newtonian fluid, 75–76, 191
Newtonian, 118
nonlinear model, 133

O
optimal radius, 164
optimal, 162–163, 198
optimization, 161, 254
optimize IABP, 259
optimizing, 164
optimum rate of energy, 165
optimum, 163
oscillometric measurement, 5
oscillometric method, 215–216
oxygen, 32–33, 190
oxygenation, 35

P
partial pressure, 32
peripheral resistance, 7, 9, 125, 184,
196
peripheral vascular resistance, 20
phase constant, 91
phase contrast magnetic resonance
imaging, 9, 88, 223
phase velocities, 101, 174, 201
photoplethysmograph, 219
pi-numbers, 44, 47
Poiseuille equation, 65, 67, 69
Poiseuille flow, 78
Poiseuille's formula, 197

Poiseuille's law, 161
Poisson ratio, 29, 50, 228
pop-test, 208, 210–211
potential energy, 70
power, 163
preload, 231, 237
pressure and flow relations, 118
pressure gradient, 43, 66–68, 114, 178, 193
pressure pulse, 218
pressure transducer, 205
pressure-compliance loop, 135
pressure-dependence of compliance, 181
pressure-dependent arterial compliance, 247
pressure-dependent compliance, 131–132, 134, 246
pressure-diameter relations, 53
pressure-diameter, 55
pressure-flow relation, 6, 191, 202
pressure-volume relation, 235, 245
pressure-volume relationship, 236
pressure-volume, 130–132, 163
propagation constant, 99
pulmonary arterial system, 82
pulmonary circulation, 5
pulsatile flow, 204
pulse pressure, 5, 80, 102, 105, 107, 173, 198, 204,
pulse transit time, 91, 219
pulse transmission efficiency, 12
pulse transmission, 151, 158, 180, 198–199
pulse wave propagation, 90, 99, 117
pulse wave reflection, 102
pulse wave transmission, 8
pulse wave velocity, 7, 12, 25, 28, 47–48, 88, 91–92, 101, 115, 122, 156, 174–175, 181–182, 199–200, 219, 245
pulse waveform analysis, 79

R
radial arterial pulse, 112
radial arteries, 1, 19, 217–218
radial pulse, 97, 217
radial strain, 27–28
radial, 206
ratio, 30
Rayleigh indices, 46
red blood cells, 35–37, 76, 187
reflected waves, 110
reflecting sites, 113
reflection coefficient, 108–109, 111
repeated and multi-site reflections, 86
repeated reflections, 113
reservoir function, 6
reservoir property, 167
resonance frequency, 209
resonant frequencies, 211
Reynolds number, 47–48, 77, 174, 191
right atrial pressure, 170, 231
right atrium, 172
right ventricle, 2, 15, 82, 172

S
servo-controlled micropipette device, 198
shear stress, 75–76, 147–148, 150–151, 204
similarity criteria, 46
sites of reflections, 81
sliding filament hypothesis, 233
Sliding Filament Theory, 232
smooth muscle, 3, 24, 26, 29–30, 41, 89, 120, 168, 183, 187, 192, 198
space-filling, 141
spring-dashpot, 55–56
Starling, 3, 173
Starling's hypothesis, 192
Starling's Law of the Heart, 237

Starling's law, 170
steady flow, 65–66, 84, 179, 191, 204
stenosis, 9, 70, 150–151, 237
Stewart-Hamilton principle, 225
storage property, 125
storage reservoir, 168
strain gages, 227
strain, 27
stress relaxation, 51, 55
stress-strain relation, 194–195
stress-strain, 49
stroke volume, 6, 82, 235–237
stroke work, 237
Swan-Ganz catheter, 206
systole, 2, 48, 79
systolic pressure, 80, 214

T
taper factor, 22
tapering, 10, 21, 81
tensile strain, 25
tensile stress, 25
tension-length relationship, 233
thermodilution, 225–227
thin wall, 28, 50
thin-walled vessels, 169
thin-walled, 19, 117, 169
three-point pressure method, 99
time constant, 127
time domain, 87–88, 103
time-varying compliance, 243, 246, 258
tonometer, 96, 173, 217
topology, 201
total peripheral resistance, 13, 90
transfer function, 94, 97, 112
transmission line theory, 113
transmission lines, 129
transmural pressures, 29–30, 50, 151, 173, 179–180, 193, 195, 216

tunica intima, 24
tunica media, 24, 26

U
ultrasonic dimension gages, 228
ultrasonic dimension gauges, 253
ultrasound dimension gages, 231
ultrasound Doppler, 220, 222
ultrasound echocardiograph, 88
ultrasound, 221

V
vascular branching, 12, 23, 81, 137–138
vascular hypertrophy, 26, 28
vascular impedance, 12, 62, 84–85, 95, 109, 152
vascular networks, 141
vascular stiffness, 12, 25, 28, 30, 94, 107, 135, 219
vascular tree, 4–5, 18, 21
vascular waterfall, 176
vasoconstriction, 3, 38, 41, 90, 103–104, 109–110
vasodilation, 90, 103–104, 107, 109–110, 135, 204
vasomotion, 188
velocity gradient, 66–67
velocity profiles, 67–69, 78, 116, 222
venous pooling, 173
venous return, 19, 167–170
ventricle-arterial system coupling, 245
ventricular ejection, 229–231, 257
viscoelastic material, 51
viscoelastic properties, 9, 100
viscoelasticity, 55
viscosities of the blood, 9

viscous modulus, 53–54
Voigt model, 55, 123
Voigt, 56
volume regulation, 239

W
wall thickness-to-radius, 30
wall thickness, 28
wall thickness-to-radius ratio, 25, 41,
  101, 158, 168
water-hammer formula, 88, 103,
  154, 156
wave reflection sites, 112

wave reflections, 12, 82–83, 90,
  96, 98, 105, 112, 152, 180, 245
wave separation method, 103
William Harvey, 2
Windkessel model, 7, 87, 125, 128,
  258
Windkessel, 82, 124, 130
Womersley's number, 156, 191
Womersley's parameter, 120–121

Y
Young's modulus of elasticity, 7,
  25–26, 49, 115, 207